THE EFFECTS OF DRUGS ON COMMUNICATION DISORDERS

Clinical Competence Series

Series Editor
Robert T. Wertz, Ph.D.

Effects of Drugs on Communication Disorders
Deanie Vogel, Ph.D, and John E. Carter, M.D.

Right Hemisphere Communication Disorders:
Therapy and Management
Connie A. Tompkins, Ph.D.

Manual of Articulation and Phonological Disorders:
From Infancy Through Adulthood
Ken M. Bleile, Ph.D.

Videoendoscopy: From Velopharynx to Larnyx
Michael P. Karnell, Ph.D.

Manual of Voice Treatment: Pediatrics Through Geriatrics
Moya L. Andrews, Ed.D., CCC-SLP

Clinical Manual of Laryngectomy and
Head and Neck Cancer Rehabilitation
Janina K. Casper, Ph.D., and Raymond H. Colton, Ph.D.

Sourcebook for Medical Speech Pathology
Lee Ann C. Golper, Ph.D., CCC-SLP

THE EFFECTS
of
DRUGS
on
COMMUNICATION
DISORDERS

Deanie Vogel, Ph.D.
Audiology and Speech Pathology Service
Department of Veterans Affairs Medical Center
Reno, Nevada

Department of Speech Pathology and Audiology
University of Nevada School of Medicine
Reno, Nevada

John E. Carter, M.D.
Division of Neurology, Department of Medicine
University of Texas Health Science Center
San Antonio, Texas

SINGULAR PUBLISHING GROUP, INC.
SAN DIEGO, CALIFORNIA

Published by Singular Publishing Group, Inc.
4284 41st Street
San Diego, California 92105-1197

©1995 by Singular Publishing Group, Inc.

Typeset in 10/12 Times by So Cal Graphics
Printed in the United States of America by BookCrafters
Figures in Chapter 1 by Nick Lang, Copyright ©1994 UTHSCSA

Library of Congress Cataloging-in-Publication Data

Vogel, Deanie
    The effects of drugs on communication disorders / Deanie Vogel, John E. Carter
      p. cm.—(Clinical competence series)
    Includes bibliographical references and index.
    ISBN 1-56593-072-X
    1. Language disorders—Chemotherapy. 2. Speech disorders—Chemotherapy.
3. Drugs—Side effects. I. Carter, John E. II. Title. III. Series
    [DNLM: 1. Communicative Disorders—drug therapy. 2. Drug Therapy—
adverse effects. WL 340.2 V878e 1994]
RC423.V644 1994
616.85'5061—dc20
DNLM/DLC
for Library of Congress   94-32171
                                                  CIP

CONTENTS

FOREWORD

com•pe•tence (kom'pə təns)   n.   The state or quality of being properly or well qualified; capable.

Clinicians crave competence. They pursue it through education and experience, through emulation and innovation. Some are more successful than others in attaining what they seek. This book, *The Effects of Drugs on Communication Disorders*, by Dr. Deanie Vogel, a speech-language pathologist, and Dr. Jack Carter, a neurologist, demonstrates how interdisciplinary collaboration can benefit us and our patients. It is one of several in the Singular Clinical Competence Series, and like the others, it is designed to move each of us further along the path that leads to clinical competence. Drs. Vogel and Carter unravel the mystery that may result from the interaction of medical and behavioral managements. They do that by telling us how drugs affect the nervous system and influence behavior. A variety of disorders are described, and specific pharmacological treatments for each are listed, including their desired effects and their possible side effects. Thus clinicians can obtain, initially, an overview of how drugs work; which drugs may be prescribed for which disorders; and how specific drugs may improve communication or, in some instances, make it worse. Subsequently, this book will serve as a reference to be consulted for application with specific patients. Mastering the contents permits speech-language pathologists to participate more effectively in their patients' entire management—behavioral and medical. Essentially, knowing about drug effects and using that knowledge in practice elevates Speech-Language Pathology beyond just being another one of the "therapies." Your attention to what Drs. Vogel and Carter provide indicates your competence and your effort to improve it, because competent clinicians seek competence as much for what it demands as for what it promises.

Robert T. Wertz, Ph.D.
Series Editor

PREFACE

This is a book about prescription drugs and their use with patients who suffer neurogenic or psychogenic communication disorders. It was written for speech-language pathologists who work in medical centers, rehabilitation clinics, private practice, public schools; any setting in which drug therapy may influence a client's communication.

Before beginning, we asked several of our speech-language pathology colleagues if they thought a book about drugs written specifically for speech-language clinicians was needed. Unanimously, they answered, "Yes." This opinion was shared by Rosenfield (1991), a physician, who wrote: "By knowing the possible effects of medical management, the informed speech-language clinician may participate more effectively in the monitoring of symptomatic changes or side effects that may be related to a particular pharmacologic regimen."

When asked for suggestions regarding content, all those questioned agreed it would be necessary to present information about how and why certain drugs work and the scientific bases of neuropharmacology. All mentioned the importance of listing the desired and possible adverse effects of drugs. We attempted to incorporate the suggestions of our colleagues. We discuss the underlying neurologic and psychiatric diseases and conditions most likely to be encountered by speech-language pathologists and the medicines currently and most commonly used to treat the disorders. Frequently, however, new drugs are approved for use, and drugs in use are withdrawn. Therefore, current, up-to-the-minute information is not always available.

Usually, the decision to approve or withdraw a drug is based on results of new investigations. Because reports of new discoveries in drug therapies are presented to the public in a timely fashion, the speech-language pathologist is advised to keep abreast of these. Presentations through radio and television, newspapers, and news magazines can be valuable sources for speech-language clinicians because they make the clinician aware of the new discoveries to which their clients and their caregivers may have been exposed. For a discussion of how new discoveries in medical management are communicated to the lay public, *see* Lozano (1991).

For information concerning topics or drugs not outlined in this book, clinicians may consult the current *Physicians' Desk Reference* or other drug manuals written specifically for physicians or nurses and available in most medical libraries.

This volume is intended to serve as a reference book and a stimulus for questions speech-language clinicians may want to ask physicians. For example, questions may arise about a specific drug prescribed for a given patient or for a patient with a specific diagnosis. The book is organized to present the causes and symptoms of a disorder, the associated symptoms and signs of communication impairment, a listing of agents used to treat the disorder, and the desired and undesirable effects of the drugs. The effects of the drug on communication follow and, finally, alternatives to medical management are discussed.

To use the book, the clinician is encouraged to look up the communication disorder of interest; check the description, causes, and common symptoms of the underlying disease or condition; check the associated speech, language, and voice symptoms; note the drugs most commonly prescribed; and consider the drugs' effects. The **Appendix** contains abbreviations of terms associated with prescription drugs and their definitions and is preceded by a Glossary of terms related to medical conditions and management.

We wish to acknowledge Robert T. Wertz, Series Editor, who conceived the idea of a book about drug therapy written specifically for speech-language pathologists. To Robin Brown who discovered and shared with us many of the references and articles used in writing this book, we are truly grateful. Also, we thank Steven Rubin, M.D., Chief, Psychiatry Service, Department of Veterans Affairs Medical Center in Reno, Nevada, for the many discussions about psychiatry, in general, and medical management of psychiatric symptoms, in particular. Finally, we acknowledge Nick Lang who drew the figures that appear in Chapter 1. This volume is meant to be a convenient and valuable reference that will enhance communication among speech-language clinicians and health care professionals with whom they share patients. We believe that the information in this book will lead to improved quality of care for the person who really matters—the communicatively disordered individual.

Deanie Vogel, Ph.D.
John E. Carter, M.D.

Recommended Readings

Lozano, R. (1991). Comanagement of disordered speech motor control: The roles of the neurologist and the speech pathologist. In D. Vogel & M. P. Cannito, (Eds.), *Treating disordered speech motor control: For Clinicians by clinicians* (Vol. 6., pp. 17-41). Austin, TX: Pro-Ed.

Rosenfield, D. B. (1991). Pharmacologic approaches to speech motor disorders. In D. Vogel & M. P. Cannito, (Eds.), *Treating disordered speech motor control: For Clinicians by clinicians* (Vol. 6., pp. 111-152). Austin, TX: Pro-Ed.

Vogel, D. (Ed). (1992). Drug treatment issues. Special Interest Division 2, *Neurophysiology and Neurogenic Speech and Language Disorders. Newsletter, 2,* (2). (Available from American Speech-Language Hearing Association, Rockville, MD.)

DEDICATION

This book is dedicated first, to Deanie Vogel, who taught me not to underestimate either the interest of speech-language pathologists in the effects of drugs on communication, or the value of the speech-language pathologist's interactions with physicians and patients. Second, I dedicate this book to the reader, as I think it should be for all books, especially when it is a first effort in the field. It is my hope that this book will be helpful to speech-language pathologists, and that its readers will let us know how to improve it in subsequent editions to even better serve their needs.

J.E.C.

To Jack Carter for convincing me that a speech-language pathologist and a physician can work together with mutual respect and admiration for each other's talents, and that they can take off and soar in new directions

and

To Arnie, who was the wind beneath my wings.

D.V.

CHAPTER

1

Basics of Neuroscience and Neuropharmacology

An understanding of brain anatomy and the physiology of neurons is necessary to appreciate the effects of drugs on communication and its disorders. Neuropharmacology is defined as the use of chemical compounds to modify the behavior of neurons and brain. Therefore, some knowledge of neurochemistry is important to understand the effects of drugs. This chapter describes how and why drugs work. It includes a review of the anatomic organization of the brain, a description of the physiology and behavior of neurons, and a discussion of neuropharmacology.

I. ANATOMY OF THE NERVOUS SYSTEM

A. Spinal Cord and Brain Stem

The lowest levels of motor and sensory processing occur in the **spinal cord** and **brainstem**.

1. **Primitive nervous systems** consist of collections of neurons that have no apparent order or organization. These neurons exist in the brain as a small amount of gray matter adjacent to the ventricular system known as the *reticular activating system*. They provide several functions that are basic necessities for all animals including **arousal** and **breathing.**

2. More **complex nervous systems** contain groups of neurons that relate to specific activities.

   a. **Spinal Cord.**

      A cross section of the spinal cord is shown in Figure 1–1. The **anterior horn** is a column of gray matter that runs the length of the spinal cord. It contains the **anterior horn cells** that provide innervation to the muscles of the body. Neurons that process sensory information are located outside the spinal cord in the **dorsal root ganglia** and in a column of neurons in the posterior part of the spinal cord. Motor reflexes such as the knee jerk are elicited at this level of the nervous system by the interaction of neurons in these two divisions of the spinal cord. All nerve fibers traveling along the spinal cord are wrapped around the anterior and posterior horns.

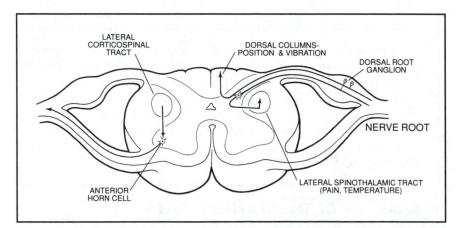

Figure 1–1.   A cross section of the spinal cord. The posterior or dorsal columns are closest to the surface of the back, receive sensory information from the sensory nerve roots (dorsal roots), and carry sensory information to the thalamus and other central nervous system structures. Other sensory fibers are present in the lateral spinal cord. Descending motor fibers in the lateral spinal cord and the anterior or ventral spinal cord synapse with the anterior horn cells in the anterior horn. The anterior horn cells are the final pathway to the muscles of the body. (Neurophysiology Study Guide, Division of Neurology, The University of Texas Health Science Center at San Antonio, copyright 1994, reproduced with permission.)

b. Brainstem.

In the brainstem, additional fiber tracts come and go from the **cerebellum.** Here, in the brainstem, specialized sensory organs begin to form their own groups of cells. Thus, the columnar organization of the spinal cord is interrupted, and cells are grouped into *nuclei.*

(1) The brainstem is divided into three structures: the **medulla,** inferiorly, the **pons,** and the **midbrain,** superiorly.

(2) Nuclei in the brainstem control muscles related to speech, chewing, facial expression, and eye movements. Sensory nuclei mediate taste, hearing, vestibular function for balance, and tactile sensation on the face.

(3) Additional nuclei coordinate visual input, vestibular input from the perception of body motion by the inner ear, and sensory information from the joints and muscles to produce smooth movements.

B. Thalamus and Basal Ganglia

The **thalamus** and the **basal ganglia** contain larger groups of neurons that have specific functions. (See Figures 1–2a & 1–2b). These structures are large, well organized, and possess their own groupings of neurons, dividing them into individual nuclei.

1. **The thalamus is divided into nuclei** according to their input and the direction of their output to the cerebral hemispheres. Thalamic nuclei receive incoming sensory information from the eyes, ears, and extremities. Much of this information is relayed to specific areas of the cerebral hemispheres where it is processed and sensations are appreciated. Some thalamic nuclei receive information from the cerebellum, the basal ganglia, and the cerebral cortex, and contribute to movement.

2. The **basal ganglia** operate with the cerebral cortex, thalamus, and cerebellum to control movement. Basal ganglia are particularly important for the initiation and smoothness of movements, especially learned, automatic movements. We can rise from a chair and walk across a room without attending to *how* we move because our basal ganglia perform these movements, leaving us free to think about what we intend to do next.

Divisions of the basal ganglia include the **striatum** (the **caudate** and the **putamen),** the **globus pallidus** and the **substantia nigra** (at the junction of the midbrain and the cerebral hemispheres), and the **subthalamic nucleus.**

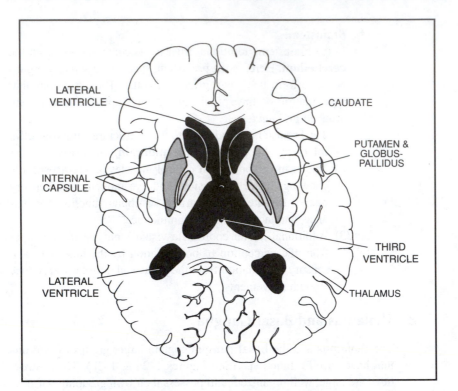

Figure 1–2a.   An axial section of the cerebral hemispheres illustrating deep structures of the brain as seen from the top of the head. The frontal lobe is shown at the top, the occipital lobe at the bottom. The temporal and parietal lobes are shown laterally. The basal ganglia are the caudate, putamen, and globus pallidus. Anteriorly, the caudate is separated from the putamen and globus pallidus by the internal capsule. The internal capsule is carrying fibers from the primary motor cortex destined for the cranial nerve nuclei of the brainstem and the anterior horn cells of the spinal cord. Additional portions of the internal capsule separate the putamen and globus pallidus from the thalamus, posteriorly. (Neurophysiology Study Guide, Division of Neurology, The University of Texas Health Science Center at San Antonio, reproduced with permission.)

C. Cerebral Hemispheres

The cerebral hemispheres make up the most visible part of the brain. Figures 1–3a and 1–3b show the cerebral hemispheres. Like the right hemisphere, the surface of the left hemisphere consists of a convoluted ribbon of gray matter that contains billions of neurons that are organized in seven layers. Beneath the cerebral cortex is a large mass of white matter made up of axons operating between the cortex and thalamus and the basal ganglia. The cerebral hemispheres are divided into areas with specific functions.

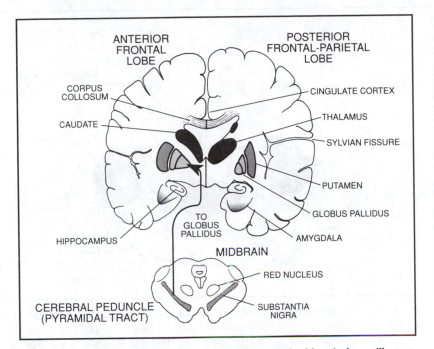

Figure 1–2b.   A frontal or coronal section of the cerebral hemispheres illustrating the basal ganglia and thalamus. On the left a section through the frontal lobe is depicted where only the basal ganglia are seen. The substantia nigra in the midbrain appears below with its projection to the globus pallidus. On the right is a section more posteriorly through the thalamus, again, separated from the putamen and globus pallidus by the internal capsule. Part of the limbic system (*see* Figure 1–4), the hippocampus and the amygdala are seen in the medial temporal lobe. (Neurophysiology Study Guide, Division of Neurology, The University of Texas Health Science Center at San Antonio, reproduced with permission.)

1. The **frontal lobes** make up nearly half of the cerebral hemispheres and lie behind the forehead and over the eyes.

    a. **The anterior frontal lobes (prefrontal area)** are responsible for conscious thought; planning for the future; understanding cause and effect; and inhibiting, delaying, or foregoing actions that will have an adverse effect at a later time.

    b. In the posterior part of the frontal lobes, just anterior to the central sulcus, is the **primary motor cortex (motor strip).** Fibers from the cells of the primary motor cortex travel directly to the brainstem motor nuclei and the anterior horn cells to produce movement.

    c. The **association motor cortex** is located between the primary motor cortex and the prefrontal area. It is thought to be impor-

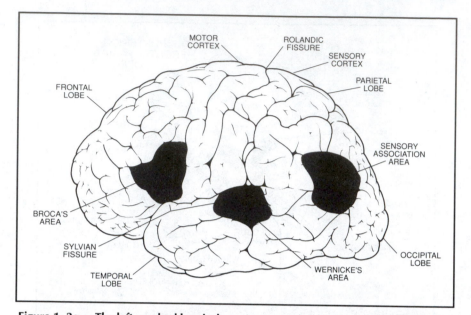

Figure 1–3a.   The left cerebral hemisphere. Important landmarks are the Rolandic fissure, the dividing line between the frontal and parietal lobes. The primary motor cortex forming the pyramidal tracts is immediately anterior to the Rolandic fissure. The primary sensory cortex receiving tactile sensory input from the spinal cord and brainstem via the thalamus is immediately posterior to the Rolandic fissure. The frontal lobe is the largest single lobe of the brain. Anterior to the motor cortex are other motor areas in the motor association cortex, and, in front of those are areas thought to be concerned with planning and emotion. The occipital lobe is a visual processing area. The primary auditory cortex is not visible on the surface of the hemisphere but lies deep inside the Sylvian fissure adjacent to Wernicke's area. The sensory association cortex at the junctions of the parietal, temporal, and occipital lobes is important for integrating and manipulating inputs of differing sensory modalities, for example, language in the left hemisphere. (Neurophysiology Study Guide, Division of Neurology, The University of Texas Health Science Center at San Antonio, reproduced with permission.)

tant in planning and in processing motor output. In addition, it has a strong connection to the basal ganglia. Broca's area, the center for motor programming of speech articulation movements, is located in this region of the left frontal lobe.

2. The **parietal lobes** lie posterior to the frontal lobes and receive all incoming tactile sensation from the skin. The parietal lobe also is important in appreciating joint and muscle position sense. The **primary sensory cortex** (somesthetic area, sensory strip), located in the anterior part of the parietal lobe, provides sensory information and acts in conjunction with the motor cortex in the frontal lobe to carry out movements. Knowledge of where a body part is located is provided by the parietal lobe and is required to achieve appropriate movement.

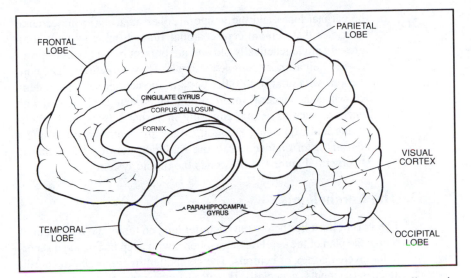

Figure 1–3b. A medial view of the right cerebral hemisphere. The corpus callosum is a large white matter structure that carries axons from one hemisphere to the other to integrate the two sides of the brain. The shaded areas are the cortical areas associated with the limbic system that lies deep to the cortex. The limbic system is illustrated in Figure 1–4. The fornix is part of the limbic system. (Neurophysiology Study Guide, Division of Neurology, The University of Texas Health Science Center at San Antonio, reproduced with permission.)

3. The **temporal lobes** are important for processing and receptive language. The **auditory association area** (Wernicke's area), located in the left temporal lobe, is necessary for the development and use of language.

4. The **occipital lobes** are located in the most posterior area of the hemispheres. The processing of visual information takes place here. Information from the left half of the visual environment registers in the **primary visual cortex** in the right hemisphere, and, conversely, information from the right half of the visual environment registers in the left hemisphere. More complex information is drawn from visual stimuli to allow perception of meaningful objects. Anteriorly, in the occipital lobe, other behaviors occur: for example, reading in the left hemisphere and recognizing faces or interpreting emotional expressions in the right hemisphere.

5. At the junction of the parietal, temporal, and occipital lobes is the **sensory association cortex.** Here, the brain makes associations: for example, associations among the visual concept of an apple, its written name, its spoken name, and the sounds of an apple being eaten.

6. **The limbic system** is a group of structures found on the medial wall of each hemisphere. It circles from the frontal lobes through

the parietal lobes and the temporal lobes adjacent to the cerebral ventricles that contain cerebrospinal fluid. Limbic system structures are phylogenetically old and are present in the brains of primitive as well as more complex animals. These structures share connections with almost all other parts of the central nervous system. Known as the **visceral brain,** the limbic system is concerned with functions such as eating, engaging in sexual activity, and experiencing and expressing emotion. Many psychotropic drugs affect neurons in or connecting to the limbic system (see Psychiatric Disorders). Figure 1–4 illustrates the limbic system.

D. The Cerebellum

The cerebellum lies below the occipital lobe on top of the brainstem. It shares the plan of the cerebral hemispheres with deep nuclei and a superficial layered cortex of neurons. The cerebellum is important in coordinated movements, especially in willed movements that require some precision, for example, reaching for an object or shooting a basketball into a hoop.

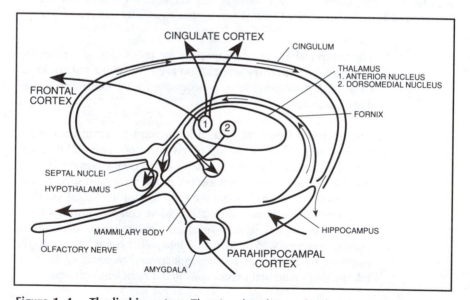

Figure 1–4.   The limbic system. The cingulum lies under the cingulate cortex. The fornix is illustrated in this figure. This circuit and its projections to and from the overlying cortex are important in emotion and for learning and memory. The arrows indicate the predominant direction of impulses flowing along a given structure. (Neurophysiology Study Guide, Division of Neurology, The University of Texas Health Science Center at San Antonio, reproduced with permission.)

E. The Hypothalamus

The hypothalamus and the autonomic nervous system regulate critical, vegetative activities such as appetite, water and electrolyte balance, temperature maintenance, and hormone production. The **hypothalamus** lies superior to the frontal lobes in the midline, adjacent to the third ventricle, and just posterior to the optic nerves. The hypothalamus directs the pituitary gland to secrete hormones and influences the autonomic nervous system.

F. Autonomic Nervous System

Divisions of the autonomic nervous system are the **sympathetic** and the **parasympathetic** systems.

1. The **sympathetic** nervous system prepares an organism for coping with stress. In a stressful situation, the pupils dilate and blood pressure, pulse, and respiration increase. As blood flow is directed to the brain and muscles, functions, for example, digestion, that are not immediately critical in a stressful situation are inhibited as blood flow is directed away from the organs that are not needed to react to stress.

   a. Neurotransmitters, for example, **epinephrine** and **norepinephrine,** produce sympathetic effects. More will be written about neurotransmitters in subsequent sections.

   b. Drugs such as **amphetamine** or **ephedrine** act to produce the same effects as the sympathetic nervous system. They are called **sympathomimetic;** because they mimic the sympathetic system. Drugs that block this response are called **sympatholytic.**

2. The **parasympathetic** system produces effects opposite to those of the sympathetic system. Relaxation—resulting in decreased pulse rate, blood pressure, and breathing rate and producing a feeling of well-being—is a function of the parasympathetic system. Relaxation techniques attempt to increase the response of the parasympathetic system and inhibit the response of the sympathetic system. Drugs may be **parasympathomimetic** or **parasympatholytic.**

Many drugs used in neuropharmacology produce side effects that affect autonomic function. Chemicals in the drugs may be identical to those **natural** neurotransmitters in the autonomic nervous system.

II. NEUROPHYSIOLOGY: NEURONS, AXONS, SYNAPSES, AND NEUROTRANSMITTERS

> The brain is made up of billions of neurons. How *individual* neurons work is fairly well understood. Thus, modifying the behavior of groups of neurons to alter brain function is possible. Exactly how *groups* of neurons interact to produce a functioning nervous system is still a mystery, especially for activities such as memory, language, and cognition.

A. The Neuron

The **neuron** is the functional unit of the brain and is designed to process information. A particular neuron receives signals from hundreds to thousands of other neurons and, in turn, sends its signal to many other neurons. A myriad of metabolic activities occurs in the neuron including the manufacture of energy substrate and protein molecules. These activities accomplish everything from repairing the cell wall, serving as enzymes for metabolic activities, and acting as neurotransmitters for signaling other cells. The majority of these cellular, metabolic activities are shared by all cells in the body. **Neurotransmission**, the unique property of neurons, provides the best opportunity for modulating neuronal function pharmacologically.

1. The **neuron cell body** manufactures all chemical substances needed to perform the neuron's function. It contains the nucleus and other structures necessary to produce energy and manufacture proteins and other chemical substances needed for the neuron to function and survive.

2. As shown in Figure 1–5, neurons communicate via their **dendrites**, **axons**, and **synapses**.

   a. **Dendrites** are multiple extensions of the cell body that receive neuronal impulses from other neurons. Some neurons have many dendrites that branch extensively and enable the neuron to receive information from many other neurons. Other neurons have only a few dendrites.

   b. The **axon** is a single, tubular extension from the cell body and is the pathway along which nerve impulses are sent to other neurons. After it leaves the cell body, the axon may branch

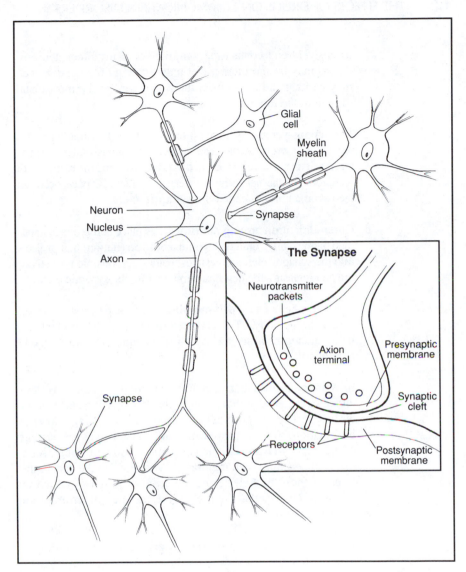

Figure 1–5. Neuronal interactions. The neuron cell body and its dendrites receive input from other neurons. Neurons send their messages to other neurons via axons. Axons are sheathed in myelin produced by glial cells called oligodendroglia. Another group of glial cells, astrocytes, not depicted in this illustration, provide the structural framework that supports the nerve cells and oligodendroglia. The inset shows a synapse—the connection between the axon of one neuron and the cell body or dendrites of another neuron—where neurotransmission occurs. Chemicals called neurotransmitters are released from the axon into the synapse where they interact with receptors on the postsynaptic cell membrane to stimulate or inhibit electrical activity in the next neuron. Details about receptors, their channels and interactions of chemicals with them are discussed in the text and are shown in Figures 1–6, 1–7 and 1–8. (Neurophysiology Study Guide, Division of Neurology, The University of Texas Health Science Center at San Antonio, reproduced with permission.)

extensively and contact the dendrites of many other neurons. Axons may be short and travel only a few millimeters, or they may be long and travel from the spinal cord to the most distal muscle in the foot.

c. The **synapse** connects an axon to a dendrite. It is made up of a presynaptic *membrane*, from which chemicals called **neurotransmitters** are released; a **postsynaptic membrane**, with receptors for the neurotransmitters; and a small space between the two membranes called the **synaptic cleft**.

d. **Communication among neurons** takes place across the synapse or synaptic cleft. Contained within a **bouton** (button) that projects into the synaptic cleft are vesicles that are responsible for activating and releasing the neurotransmitters into the synaptic cleft.

3. The neuron is bound by a **cell membrane** that separates it from all other cells in the body. The nerve cell membrane allows electrical signaling among neurons, and thus makes communication among neurons possible.

a. **Ions** are molecules that carry one or more extra electrons. Ions either are negatively charged or, if they are missing one or more electrons, they are positively charged. The signaling (flow) of information from one nerve cell to another involves the passage of electrically charged chemical particles (ions) through separate channels in the cell membrane. Variations in the concentrations of these particles generate a nerve impulse, called an *action potential*, that facilitates the transfer of information among neurons.

b. A cell membrane is **selectively permeable** to specific elements. Although water can flow in and out of cell membranes, not all chemicals can cross all membranes. Ions can cross membranes with varying degrees of ease.
   (1) The ions important for neuronal signaling are **potassium**, **sodium**, **calcium**, and **chloride**. Differences in the permeability of the cell membrane for two of these ions (potassium = high permeability, sodium = low permeability) create a **resting electrical potential** across the cell membrane.
   (2) Each ion passes in or out of the neuron across the cell membrane through its **channel**. Channels are complex molecules that may be opened or closed to ions and, therefore, are referred to as **"gates."** When the channel is open, the ions can flow to one side or the other. When the cell membrane is inactive and the **resting membrane potential** is established, the channel is closed.

(3) A **voltage-gated channel** shown in Figure 1–6 allows for the **movement** of ions. When the voltage reaches a certain level, the channel opens, and the ions can flow across the cell membrane. Any given channel allows the passage of only one type of ion. There is a voltage-gated channel specific to every ion that is considered to be important in neurophysiology. Some channels are opened when the voltage in the adjacent cell membrane decreases. Others are opened when another molecule, a *neurotransmitter*, is added to change the configuration in the cell wall (see Figure 1–7).

(4) To generate a nerve impulse, the nerve cell membrane must be **depolarized**, that is, there must be an electrical charge across the cell membrane. Depolarization begins when a sodium channel across the membrane opens briefly and sodium ions pass through it into the cell.

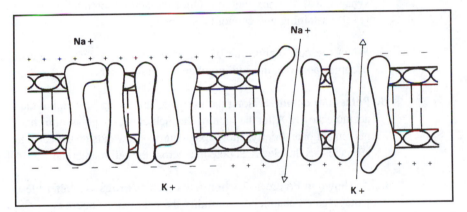

Figure 1–6.   Voltage-gated ion channels in the cell wall of an axon. Ion channels are of two types—chemically-gated and voltage-gated. Here, channels allowing sodium or potassium to cross the membrane are shown closed when the nerve cell membrane is polarized—usually to about –70 millivolts inside the cell. There is a positive charge outside the cell wall where the concentration of sodium (Na+) is high and negative charge inside the cell where the potassium (K+) concentration is high. When the cell wall depolarizes partially to a threshold value of approximately 40 millivolts, the channels open, and allow complete depolarization to occur. Because electrical charges move toward opposite charges, the cell membrane adjacent to the depolarized area will lose some of its electrical charge. The next event to occur after that depicted in the illustration will be the movement of the ions on the cell membrane toward the right where depolarization has occurred. Threshold will be reached, the closed channels will open, and depolarization will continue along the cell membrane, producing an action potential. The channels will close when the cell membrane has been completely depolarized. The sodium channel opens first and produces depolarization. The potassium channel opens later and closes later than the sodium channel, and pushes positive ions outside to reestablish the negative charge inside the cell. (Neurophysiology Study Guide, Division of Neurology, The University of Texas Health Science Center at San Antonio, reproduced with permission.)

B. The Synapse

All signaling begins and ends at the *synapse*.

1. To generate a nerve impulse (action potential), the cell membrane of the axon must be depolarized. **Sodium** channels along the axon are **voltage-gated**. These channels open if the voltage decreases to a threshold value. This occurs when the cell body and dendrites adjacent to the beginning of the axon become depolarized.

2. Once the sodium channels on the axon open, sodium enters the cell and the membrane potential reaches zero. Electrical charge flows from the adjacent axon membrane, depolarizes that section, and opens its sodium channel.

3. In this way, the action potential continues down the axon to synapse with the next neuron. Once the action potential begins, it is self-sustaining and cannot be stopped.

4. When the cell membrane of the axon reaches a zero charge or becomes positive, the sodium channels close again.

5. **Potassium channels** along the axon also are voltage-gated, but they act more slowly. After the sodium channels close, the potassium channel remain open briefly, allows potassium to flow outside the cell and reestablishes the electrical potential across the cell membrane.

6. As shown in Figure 1–7, **chemicals** such as **drugs** may alter these voltage-gated channels and modify the behavior of neurons.

   a. All neurons have the same voltage-gated channels for sodium and potassium as well as for other ions. Although chemicals, drugs, for example, may alter these channels, they can be nonselective and not affect all neurons in the same fashion. Therefore, some chemicals can become toxic rather than therapeutic.

   b. If Puffer fish, a gourmet delicacy, is not prepared carefully, the diner may ingest tetrodotoxin—a neurochemical contained in the ovaries of the fish. Tetrodotoxin disables the sodium voltage-gated channels and results in a shut-down in all neuronal activity. Similar toxins have developed in paralytic shellfish (saxotoxin), South American poisonous frogs (batrachotoxin), and North African scorpions. Serving such ill-prepared "gourmet foods" may be a "not-so-obvious" but highly successful method of eliminating one's enemies.

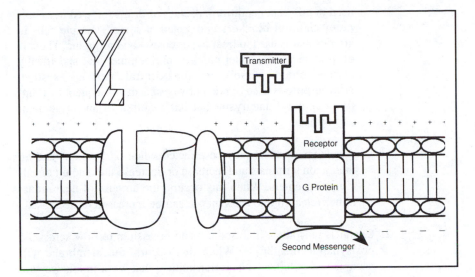

Figure 1–7.   Chemical-gated channels at a synapse. The synaptic cleft is toward the top of the illustration, and two different neurotransmitter molecules are depicted free in the cleft. Receptors are of two types. On the left is an ion channel that opens when the transmitter alters the shape of the molecule making up the receptor. In this case, the channel allowed flow of both sodium (going into the cell) and potassium (going out of the cell) and produced partial depolarization of the postsynaptic membrane. The change in voltage does not affect the channel as it does the voltage-gated channels depicted in Figure 1–6, however the channel will remain open for as long as a transmitter molecule fits into it. If the depolarization in the synapse is sufficient, an electrical charge will flow from the adjacent axon cell membrane, and voltage-gated channels there will open, initiating an action potential. Other receptors, depicted on the right, activate a metabolic system to produce an enzyme that enhances a specific metabolic activity in the cell. For example, the production of an enzyme used to manufacture a neurotransmitter may be increased and result in the presence of more neurotransmitter in the axon terminal and more effective transmission in the synapse. Because the effect is the result of this indirect process, it is referred to as a **second messenger system**. (Neurophysiology Study Guide, Division of Neurology, The University of Texas Health Science Center at San Antonio, reproduced with permission.)

7. Chemicals used for neurotransmission (**neurotransmitters**) are stored at the axon terminal inside packets called **synaptic vesicles**. If **calcium** is present inside the axon terminal, the membrane around these packets can attach to the presynaptic membrane and release the chemical into the synapse.

   a. The axon terminal contains **calcium channels** that are voltage-gated. When the action potential reaches the axon terminal, these channels open allowing calcium to enter the cell and stimulate the release of neurotransmitters into the synapse.

   b. Calcium channels have different configurations in different organs that allow site-specific **calcium channel blockers** to be used in different conditions. A class of drugs referred to as **calcium channel blockers** is directed at smooth muscle cells in arteries and is used to treat hypertension and migraine. There is even a calcium channel blocker, nimodipine, that specifically affects blood vessels in the central nervous system. **Nimodipine** is used to prevent vasospasm subsequent to a ruptured cerebral aneurysm that has resulted in an intracranial hemorrhage.

c. A calcium channel may be affected when other axons end on their axon terminals and increase or decrease the amount of calcium that enters. When this occurs, the amount of neurotransmitter released into the synapse can be increased or decreased.

2. Channels may allow both sodium and potassium to flow across the postsynaptic membrane. When this occurs, the membrane will become less polarized. Neurotransmitters that work in this way are called **excitatory**, because they attempt to initiate an action potential.

3. Channels may allow **chloride**, a negatively charged ion, to flow into the cell. This results in a greater negative charge inside the cell. Neurotransmitters that work in this way are called **inhibitory,** because they make it less likely that an action potential will occur.

4. Dendrites constantly change the electrical potential across the cell membrane. When the membrane potential change is great enough, the voltage-gated channels of the junction of the cell body and the axon will open, and an action potential will be generated and will travel down the axon.

5. Another adjacent protein in the cell wall may be activated. When this occurs, a signal is sent via a chemical reaction inside the cell to produce more of the chemical (usually the neurotransmitter) used by that cell. This action indirectly affects subsequent signaling by the receiving neuron, because the more transmitter available in the axon terminal, the more that will be released when a signal is sent.

C. Neurotransmitters and Receptors

1. **Neurotransmitters**, shown in Figure 1–8, are varied, and each one is associated with specific groups of neurons. Transmitters have been described according to how their component atoms come together to form molecules. Each neurotransmitter molecule has a

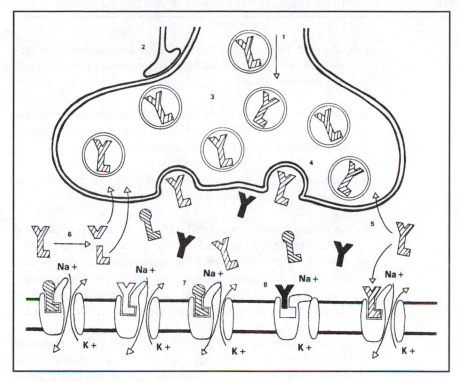

Figure 1–8. **The synapse.** The axon terminal is shown with packets of neurotransmitter. These neurotransmitters are released into the synaptic cleft where they bind with receptors on the post-synaptic membrane and open those channels to ion flow. Signal transmission between neurons can be modified best at the synapse by altering the activity of the neurotransmitter system. This is accomplished in several ways. First, the amount of neurotransmitter manufactured by the cell and sent to the axon terminal can be increased or decreased. This can be accomplished by changing the amount of precursors available to manufacture the neurotransmitter or activating enzymes that metabolize the precursor. Second, presynaptic inhibition or facilitation occurs by altering the amount of calcium allowed to enter the neuron when an action potential arrives, thus increasing or decreasing the number of neurotransmitter vesicles that can bind to the presynaptic membrane and release their transmitter into the synaptic cleft. Third, the amount of neurotransmitter stored in the axon terminal can be increased or decreased. Fourth, release of the neurotransmitter can be facilitated or inhibited at the presynaptic membrane. Fifth, after a neurotransmitter is released into the synaptic cleft, some of it is reabsorbed into the axon terminal. This absorption can be enhanced or inhibited, allowing a shorter or longer duration of action of released transmitter molecules. Sixth, neurotransmitter molecules are metabolized so they do not remain in the synaptic cleft indefinitely, thus breakdown of the molecule may be inhibited or enhanced. Seventh, a molecule similar in configuration to the neurotransmitter, an agonist, may be administered to stimulate the receptors. Eighth, a molecule that can bind with the receptor sufficiently to block the normal transmitter, but that does not alter the receptor enough to open the channel, may be administered to antagonize the action of the neurotransmitter. Most of neuropharmacology is aimed at making these alterations at the synapse to enhance or inhibit a given set of neurons and their actions. (Neurophysiology Study Guide, Division of Neurology, The University of Texas Health Science Center at San Antonio, reproduced with permission.)

17

unique shape. For example, complex neurotransmitters are three-dimensional. All are protein molecules that interact with receptors in nerve cell membranes.

2. **Receptors** are segments of the cell membrane that also are made up of complex protein molecules. When binding occurs with one of the body's neurotransmitters, one of two events may occur.

   a. The segment of the cell membrane may become permeable to ions and thus will excite or inhibit an action potential.

   b. An adjacent protein in the cell wall may become activated and send a signal via a chemical reaction inside the cell to produce more of a chemical—usually the neurotransmitter used by that cell. This action affects subsequent signaling by the receiving neuron indirectly. When a signal is sent, the more transmitter available in the axon terminal, the more that will be released.

3. A neurotransmitter molecule and its receptor have been compared to a key and lock. In this analogy, the neurotransmitter molecule is the key that fits into the receptor lock in the cell membrane. There may be a variety of neurotransmitters with similar enough structures that can attract, fit, and activate a given receptor. The "winner" neurotransmitter will be the one whose shape conforms most closely to the fit of the receptor.

   a. One neurotransmitter may compete for a receptor with other neurotransmitters that have only slightly different configurations. Furthermore, a neurotransmitter may be taken up by a certain receptor but fail to activate it at another time. How successful a given neurotransmitter will be in activating a receptor depends upon other neurotransmitters that are available at that particular time (Restak, 1994).

   b. Molecules other than the body's naturally occurring neurotransmitters may stimulate the receptors. These molecules can be medicines, referred to as **agonists**, or they can be toxins.

   c. A key may fit into a lock but fail to turn it. Similarly, neurotransmitter molecules may have similar enough shapes to bind with a receptor superficially, but they may not be similar enough to change the receptor's configuration. While this will not alter the activity, the presence of the molecule may block the effective neurotransmitter from binding with the receptor. Such medicines are called **antagonists**.

d. All chemical compounds used in the body are made from smaller basic molecules that are called **precursors**. Many, including neurotransmitters, are also metabolized or broken down; sometimes back into the original precursors and other times into other inactive compounds called **breakdown products. Enzymes** are molecules that somehow facilitate the chemical reactions but remain unchanged. Thus, they are not incorporated into the new molecule, and, therefore, can participate in the reactions repeatedly.

4. Four major types of neurotransmitters are **amino acids**; **acetylcholine**; the **monoamines** (**catecholamines** and **serotonin**); and a chemically mixed group (histamine, nitric oxide, and a group of small molecules composed of short chains of amino acids) called **neuropeptides**.

a. **Amino acids** are simple chemicals that serve as the building blocks for proteins. They are part of our diet and are present throughout the brain and the body. Several amino acids may act as neurotransmitters.

(1) **Glutamate** and **aspartate** are the most important amino acids in neurotransmission and are the primary **excitatory** messengers within the brain. These amino acids are found throughout the brain and spinal cord.

(2) GABA (**gamma-amino butyric acid**) is the most prevalent inhibitory neurotransmitter in the central nervous system. It also is found throughout the brain and spinal cord.

b. **Acetylcholine** (Ach) is localized to the several neuronal systems shown in Figure 1–9. Neurons using Ach as a transmitter are called **cholinergic**.

(1) Ach is the transmitter located at the synapse between the nerves and the muscles at the neuromuscular junctions. It is the transmitter in the parasympathetic nervous system that stimulates a variety of structures including the gastrointestinal tract.

(2) Ach is used by small "interneurons" in the basal ganglia that are important in processing and modifying signals within a small confined area of the brain.

(3) Ach is the transmitter of a group of cells deep in the cerebral hemispheres (the nucleus basalis of Meynert) and is important in memory. It may activate or arouse cortical

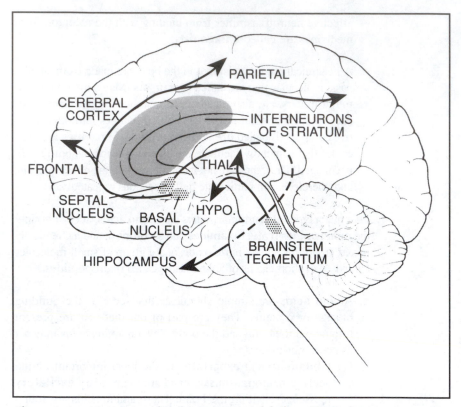

Figure 1–9.   Neurotransmitter systems: Acetylcholine. This is the neurotransmitter for many short axon interneurons within the striatum. It is also the transmitter of midline nuclear groups at the base of the brain from which there are projections to the entire cerebral cortex. This group of neurons is decreased in Alzheimer's disease. (Neurophysiology Study Guide, Division of Neurology, The University of Texas Health Science Center at San Antonio, reproduced with permission).

neuronal systems. In Alzheimer's disease, the basal nuclei degenerate. Significantly less Ach has been found in the cerebral cortex of Alzheimer's patients than in the brains of persons with no history of the disease.

  c. **Monoamines** are divided into the **catecholamines** and **serotonin**.
    (1) Catecholamines include **dopamine, norepinephrine (noradrenaline)**, and **epinephrine (adrenaline)**.
    (2) Dopamine, shown in Figure 1-10, is the inhibitory neurotransmitter used by the hypothalamus to regulate hormonal activity in the pituitary gland. It is the transmitter for two groups of neurons located in the brainstem; the substantia

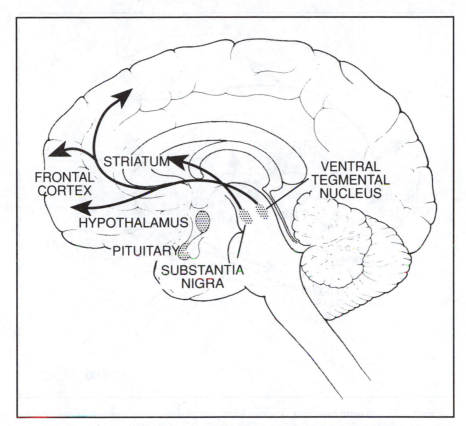

Figure 1–10.   Neurotransmitter systems: Dopamine. The dopaminergic system has three main cell groups that utilize dopamine as a neurotransmitter. The substantia nigra projects to the striatum to regulate movement. This group of dopaminergic neurons degenerates in Parkinson's disease. The ventral tegmental nucleus projects to the frontal lobes and plays a role in schizophrenia. The hypothalamus uses dopamine to regulate certain hormonal activities such as lactation. (Neurophysiology Study Guide, Division of Neurology, The University of Texas Health Science Center at San Antonio, reproduced with permission.)

nigra and the **ventral tegmental** area. The axons in the substantia nigra project to the basal ganglia and are important for movement. Neurons in the ventral tegmental area project diffusely to the frontal lobes and the limbic system and are believed to be involved in schizophrenia. In Parkinson's disease, nerve cells in the substantia nigra are lost and the result is a deficiency of dopamine.

(3) Cells using **norepinephrine**, shown in Figure 1–11, are called noradrenergic. Norepinephrine is the neurotransmitter used by a group of cells in the brainstem, the *locus ceruleus*. These cells project widely through the cerebral

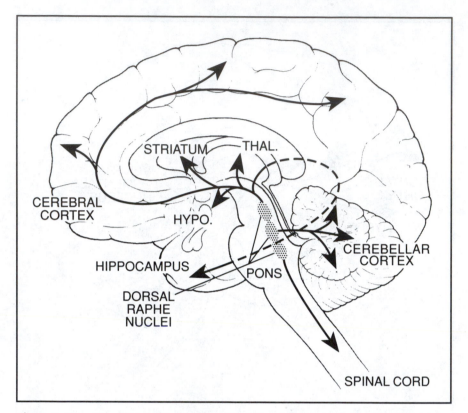

Figure 1–11.   Neurotransmitter systems: Norepinephrine. Noradrenergic cells originate in the brainstem in a group of cells called the locus ceruleus. These cells project widely to the cerebral cortex where they play a role in mood disorders and anxiety. Another group projects to the hypothalamus and is involved in regulation of the functions of the autonomic nervous system. (Neurophysiology Study Guide, Division of Neurology, The University of Texas Health Science Center at San Antonio, reproduced with permission.)

hemispheres and the spinal cord and are thought to be involved in mood disorders and anxiety.

(4) **Serotonin**, shown in Figure 1–12, is used by groups of cells located in the brainstem **(the dorsal raphe)** and projects widely throughout the brain and spinal cord. Serotonin is important in sleep-wake cycles, emotion and mood disorders, and functions mediated by the limbic system.

(5) **Epinephrine** is limited to cells in the brainstem that project to the autonomic nervous system centers.

d. **Neuropeptides** influence signaling within the brain indirectly by facilitating the action of and prolonging the response to the

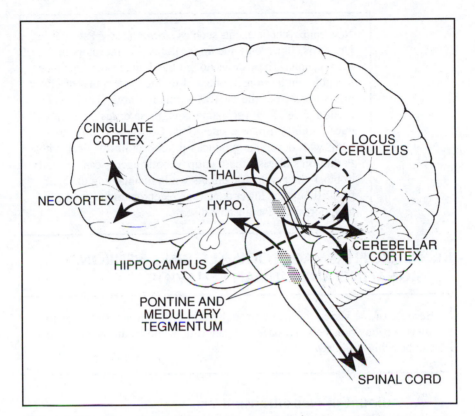

Figure 1–12.   Neurotransmitter systems: Serotonin. Serotonergic neurons are located in a group of neurons in the brainstem called the dorsal raphe nuclei and project widely throughout the central nervous system. (Neurophysiology Study Guide, Division of Neurology, The University of Texas Health Science Center at San Antonio, reproduced with permission.)

major neurotransmitters. Neuropeptides include the **endorphins—Substance P** and **Substance K**.

5. Just as a master key unlocks several different doors, one neurotransmitter can activate several different receptors. Too much dopamine (from too many activated receptors) results in hallucinations and other psychotic behaviors of schizophrenia and is seen as a complication of dopamine therapy in Parkinson's disease. Conversely, too little dopamine produces motor slowing, a symptom of dopamine *deficiency* in Parkinson's disease, and is seen as a complication of treatment for schizophrenia that utilizes dopamine blocking drugs (Posner & Raichle, 1994).

New antipsychotic agents such as *clozapine* (*see* Psychiatric Disorders) block only the *upper* dopamine receptors in the basal ganglia. These drugs do not block the lower dopamine receptors in the frontal lobe and limbic system that receive projections from the ventral tegmental area. Thus, when used in patients with schizophrenia, these drugs do not produce Parkinsonism as a side effect. Conversely, when treatment with dopamine produces psychosis in a patient with Parkinson's disease, these antipsychotic agents can be used to block the psychiatric effects while maintaining the benefit of stimulating lower dopamine receptors in the basal ganglia to treat the Parkinson's disease.

III. NEUROPHARMACOLOGY: ALTERING NEURONAL SIGNALING AND HUMAN BEHAVIOR

Because of the variety of neurotransmitters in different neuronal systems, altering behavior is best approached by altering events in the synapse. This can be achieved in several ways.

A. Amount of Neurotransmitter

The amount of neurotransmitter produced by the neurons can be altered.

1. More or less of the neurotransmitter is produced in the cell body and sent to the axon terminal.

2. Storage at the axon terminal can be changed, thereby altering the amount of the neurotransmitter available for release into the synapse upon the arrival of an action potential.

3. Many drugs deplete the stores of a neurotransmitter in the axon terminal, and, therefore, there is less drug available for release. The drug **Reserpine** depletes *noradrenergic* transmitter stores and lowers blood pressure but it also alters noradrenergic neurons in the central nervous system, producing depression as a side effect.

4. The amount of transmitter released into the synapse can be altered in the following ways:

    a. Some axons terminate on other axon terminals close to the synapse and change the amount of calcium allowed to enter the

axon terminal. Thus the binding and release of packets of neurotransmitter into the synapse is increased or decreased.

b. Other compounds may act at the presynaptic membrane to
inhibit or facilitate release of the neurotransmitter packets into
the synapse. Botulinum toxin is such a compound. It blocks the
release of acetylcholine from neurons to skeletal muscle, and
produces weakness or paralysis of the muscles (*See* Idiopathic
Speech Disorders.)

5. The reuptake of the neurotransmitter through the presynaptic membrane into the axon terminal can be changed, and allows the transmitter to remain in the synaptic cleft to stimulate the receptors for
a longer period of time.

6. The sensitivity of the postsynaptic receptor can be altered. In this
case, the receptor is blocked with a molecule that resembles the
transmitter closely enough to bind with the receptor but not closely enough to activate it. Neuroleptic medicines such as **Haldol** (*see*
Psychiatric Disorders, schizophrenia) block **dopamine** receptors.

7. The postsynaptic receptor can be stimulated directly with a compound that mimics the neurotransmitter.

IV. PHARMACOKINETICS

To be effective, a drug must be absorbed, arrive at the organ to be affected,
and be metabolized. These processes affect how a drug is prescribed, its interaction with other drugs, its duration of action, and its potential for toxicity.

A. Drug Absorption

Drug absorption depends on the route of administration, how a drug is
formulated, its molecule's size, its solubility in water and in lipids, its
resistance to breakdown in the gastrointestinal tract (GI), and the presence of food in the gastrointestinal tract.

1. Drug formulation has become quite sophisticated. Drugs may be
designed to be released slowly in the GI tract in several ways, for
example, in a slowly dissolving preparation. The drug may be
enclosed in material that allows water to enter, and a small hole is
made allowing the increasing volume of water crossing over the
membrane to squeeze the drug out.

> Slowly released medication may not be an option for everyone. For example, it is not possible to use this type of preparation with children for whom the tablets must be crushed or for the dysphagic patient who is being fed via a gastric tube.

2. To make a drug soluble in water, it may be formulated for administration in an acid or basic solution. Not all medicines formulated in such solutions can be administered by intramuscular injection. For example, **Dilantin**® (*see* Epilepsy) is formulated in a basic solution. If Dilantin® is given intramuscularly, it will form an abscess instead of being absorbed.

B. Drug Distribution

Drug distribution is influenced by several factors.

1. **Membrane permeability**. A drug must pass through all membranes between its site of administration and the organ it is to affect.

   a. Many antibiotics are readily absorbed from the GI tract but do not pass through the blood brain barrier (*see* Glossary). Thus, antibiotics are not effective for treating infections of the brain.

   b. **Benzodiazepines**, such as **Valium**® and **Ativan**® (*see* Psychiatric Disorders), are lipophilic (lipid soluble) and pass readily through the wall of the GI tract, the blood vessel walls, and the blood brain barrier.

   c. **Dopamine**, the deficient neurotransmitter in Parkinson's disease, will not cross the blood brain barrier, and, therefore, its precursor L-DOPA is given. L-DOPA crosses the blood brain barrier readily where it is metabolized to the required dopamine.

2. **Lipophilic drugs**, including many drugs active in the central nervous system, accumulate in body fat. These drug stores are released slowly. They reduce the frequency with which they must be administered but they also prolong the duration of possible overdose.

C. Drug Metabolism

Drugs are just one of many chemicals to which we are exposed. Our bodies attempt to get rid of all chemicals, usually by transforming them into more water soluble molecules that can be excreted by the kidneys.

Many drugs metabolized in the liver affect tolerance (*see* Glossary). Alcohol is an example of such a drug. People who are not used to drinking alcohol may become tipsy after a drink or two. If they consume two drinks daily for several weeks, it will require more than two drinks for them to achieve the same degree of intoxication as when they first began to drink.

D. Drug Excretion

Some drugs are metabolized unchanged, and others are metabolized to more soluble forms. Most drugs, toxins, and their metabolites are excreted in the urine and some are excreted in the feces or expired air.

E. Drug Levels

Unless given by a continuous infusion by vein, drug levels cannot be maintained at an absolutely steady state in the serum (blood) or the body. After administration, the serum level of a drug rises until, as it is absorbed, a peak level is reached. After the drug is completely absorbed, the level slowly drops to a lowest level, **the trough**, before it starts to rise with the next dose. The **half life** is the period of time it takes for the plasma level of a material to decrease by 50%. In general, the longer the half life of a drug the better, since it may be given less often. Ideally, a drug should be administered twice each half life to diminish the fluctuation between peak and trough levels. Sustained release (SR) preparations compensate for this to some degree but are slower acting.

G. Recommended Readings

Bloom, F. E., & Lazerson, A. (1988). *Brain, mind, and behavior*. New York: W. H. Freeman.

Posner, M. I., & Raichle, M. E. (1994). *Images of mind*. New York: Scientific American Library, HPHLP.

Restak, R. M. (1994). *Receptors*. New York: Bantam Books.

CHAPTER

2

Speech and Voice Specific Neurologic Disorders

This chapter covers neurologic disorders that may affect speech and voice production. For each disorder, we provide a definition and cause; discuss the general features, symptoms, and signs; describe the features, symptoms, and signs of communication impairment associated with each disorder; list pharmacologic treatment for each disorder; and discuss the influence drug treatment may have on communication.

I. PARKINSON'S DISEASE

A. Definition/Cause

1. Parkinson's disease is a **progressive movement disorder** characterized by decrease in spontaneous movement, gait difficulty, postural instability, rigidity, and resting tremor. A small group of neurons, the substantia nigra (literally, "black substance" because it contains the black pigment, melanin), is located on each side of the brain stem. These pigmented neurons degenerate and die, resulting in the decreased dopamine availability responsible for Parkinson's disease.

2. Both males and females are affected, with a **higher incidence after age 50 years.** One in 40 individuals over age 65 years is affected by Parkinson's disease. The incidence and prevalence of Parkinson's disease in persons under age 40 years appear to be increasing.

3. The **primary etiology** of Parkinson's disease has not been determined. Toxins, dietary factors, heredity, infectious processes, or a combination of these may be responsible for the degeneration or malfunction of cells in the substantia nigra.

4. Most patients in the first 50 years of this century experienced Parkinson's disease as a late complication of the world-wide encephalitis epidemic of the 1917–1918 period. There was speculation that the disease would become unusual as that group of patients grew old and died. Unfortunately, this has not happened. Now there is concern that industrialization and exposure to various man-made toxins may be a major contributing factor to the occurrence of Parkinson's disease.

B. General Features, Symptoms, and Signs

1. Symptoms were described in 1817 by Dr. James Parkinson who referred to the condition as "shaking palsy." Although Dr. Parkinson was a general practitioner, and not a specialist in neurological disorders, his description of Parkinson's disease appears to be current and completely valid today.

2. The first symptoms appear after there is at least an 80% loss of pigmented neurons with a similar decrease in dopamine availability.

3. Major features are **resting tremor, bradykinesia,** and **rigidity.** Symptoms may remain mild for a long period or may progress steadily. Eventually, the tremor spreads, and most of the muscles become rigid. The posture may be stooped, and there may be slow, jerky movements, shuffling, and unsteady gait. Facial expression may be lost, hence, the sign of **"masked facies"** is noted.

   a. **Resting tremor** is a rhythmic, to-and-fro movement of the extremity and, occasionally, the jaw. It disappears with the intentional use of the extremity and when the patient is asleep. In some patients, there is an associated action tremor present during movement.

   b. Patients with **bradykinesia** may be slow to arise from a chair, may require several small steps to turn around; may show diminished responses to events such as spilling liquids; and, in extreme cases, are unable to get up out of a chair or turn over in bed. Discontinuing an ongoing movement, such as walking, may be affected so that patients have as difficult a time stopping as they do starting to walk.

c. **Rigidity** is increased resistance to passive movements of a limb that is present throughout the range of movement. It is accentuated if the patient performs a movement with the limb opposite to the one that is being moved. In Parkinson's disease, rigidity may fluctuate during movement in a fashion that parallels the tremor, a **"cogwheel rigidity."** **Stooped posture** with **flexed arms** and **bent knees** is associated with rigidity.

d. **Depression** has been reported in approximately 30% of cases.

e. **Dysphagia** with increased oral-pharyngeal transit time and impaired airway protection has been observed.

C. Features, Symptoms, and Signs of Communication Impairment

1. The speech associated with Parkinson's disease has been described as a **hypokinetic dysarthria.** The common characteristics are short rushes of speech, monopitch, monoloudness, and reduced loudness.

2. Voice volume and speech intelligibility may deteriorate rapidly during an utterance. Vocal tremor may be present.

3. Written communication may be impaired. A common feature is **micrographia,** handwriting in which the height of the letters is small and becomes increasingly smaller as the patient writes.

4. **Dementia** with accompanying loss of communication skills has been identified.

D. Pharmacologic Treatment

Anti-Parkinson's drugs and their common side effects are shown in Table 2–1.

1. **Anticholinergic Drugs.** Initially, **anticholinergics** were the sole therapy for Parkinson's disease. These drugs were somewhat effective in alleviating tremor but had little effect on bradykinesia and

Table 2-1. Anti-Parkinson medications.

Drug	Actions	Indications	Side Effects
LEVODOPA (L-DOPA)	Converted to dopamine in CNS; supplements dopamine released by nigrostriatal neurons.	Seldom used alone; replaced by a combination of levodopa plus a peripheral decarboxylase inhibitor such as Sinemet®, Sinemet CR® (controlled release), or Prolopa®	Gastrointestinal disorder, orthostatic hypotension, arrhythmias in older patients, increased sexual activity due to action on the hypothalamus, choreiform movements, vivid dreams, hallucinations, psychosis
SINEMET® (LEVODOPA + CARBIDOPA)	Combination L-DOPA plus peripheral decarboxylase inhibitor. Decreased systemic side effects of levodopa.	Primary drug therapy for Parkinson's disease	Similar to levodopa, except considerably less systemic toxicity: dyskinesias, vivid dreams and hallucinations, psychosis. Increased sexual activity due to actions on the hypothalamus.
PROLOPA® (Benserazide + Levodopa)	Similar to Sinemet	Primary drug therapy for Parkinson's disease	Similar to Sinemet®
BROMOCRIP-TINE	Powerful dopamine agonist	Adjunct therapy to levodopa or prescribed when tolerance to levodopa develops.	Gastrointestinal disturbance, hypotension, hallucinations, confusion. Less dyskinesia than with levodopa.
PERGOLIDE®	Dopamine agonist more potent than bromocriptine	Adjunct therapy to levodopa/carbidopa	Dyskinesia, nausea, rhinitis, constipation, dizziness, hallucinations, somnolence
AMANTA-DINE®	Releases dopamine from intact nigrostriatal nerve endings.	May be used as initial therapy in mild cases. May be used as adjunctive therapy in patients experiencing on-off effect while on levodopa.	Congestive heart failure, pedal edema, urinary retention, visual hallucinations, paranoid delusions, nightmares, mania, depression.

rigidity. Therefore, as the disease progressed, patients soon became totally disabled. Today, anticholinergic medications are used primarily in early Parkinson's disease when tremor is the primary complaint. They are used as ancillary drugs but have no major role in treating the disease.

a. Commonly used anticholinergic drugs are ethopropozine **(Parsidol®), benzotropine (Cogentin®), biperiden (Akineton®),** and **trihexyphenidyl (Artane®).**

(1) **Desired effect** is relief from tremor in the initial stages of the disease.

(2) **Undesirable effects. Blurred vision, dry mouth, constipation, impaired urination,** and **nervousness** are common side effects that usually subside with continued drug use. Less common side effects are **skin rash, headache, dizziness, drowsiness, muscle cramps, indigestion,** and **gastrointestinal disturbance.** Serious adverse effects are **confusion, memory loss, agitation, auditory and visual hallucinations,** and **delusions.**

2. Levodopa; L-DOPA (Dopar®, Larodopa®), a dopamine agonist, has been the standard treatment for Parkinson's disease. Once in the central nervous system, levodopa is converted to dopamine, replacing the lost dopamine responsible for the Parkinsonian symptoms.

> Dopamine replacement was attempted initially in miners in South America who developed Parkinsonian symptoms as a result of their exposure to manganese. Although initial response to dopamine replacement was poor, when patients were given high doses a significant decrease in their symptoms was achieved. Subsequent trials with patients with Parkinson's disease proved successful.

a. Desired effects are decreased rigidity, increased facility of movement, and decrease of resting tremor.

(1) Approximately 80% of patients demonstrate initial improvement with levodopa. The dosage of the drug is gradually increased until adequate control of symptoms is achieved without unacceptable side effects.

b. Undesirable effects are **gastrointestinal disturbance, postural hypotension** (*see* Glossary), **syncope (fainting), dry mouth, blurred vision,** and **cardiac arrhythmias.** The side effects may decrease or disappear with a lower dose of levodopa.

(1) High doses result in **dyskinesias (uncontrolled involuntary movements)** that occur 20–90 minutes after the medicine is taken.

(2) **Vivid dreams** and **nightmares** may be reduced when the last dose of the day is lowered. Additional side effects are **confusion, agitation, overt hallucinations** and **psychosis;** these reverse rapidly with reduction of the dosage.

(3) Levodopa may stimulate the hypothalamus, producing **increased sexual activity.**

(4) **Depression** may become more evident when levodopa is taken as patients become more animated and expressive of their feelings.

(5) **On-off phenomenon** and **end-of-dose akinesia** both are manifested by a return of symptoms. The on-off phenomenon is not specifically related to dosage, but both the off and the end-of-dose symptoms have been linked to low plasma levels of levodopa. On-off phenomena are unpredictable episodes lasting from 30 minutes to a few hours and are characterized by a sudden **inability to move, hypertonia,** and **apprehension.** The episodes begin and terminate rapidly and without warning. Some authors believe the on-off phenomenon is related to the duration of the drug treatment and others believe duration of treatment is unrelated. About half of the patients treated for longer than 5 years experience an on-off phenomenon. Changes to smaller doses given more frequently, as often as every 2 hours, may prevent both on-off and end-of-dose effects.

3. **Levodopa** and **Peripheral Decarboxylase Inhibitors: Sinemet®, Madopar®,** and **Prolopa®.** Virtually all patients are treated with a combination of **levodopa** and a **dopa-decarboxylase inhibitor** that blocks or diminishes most of the peripheral systemic side effects of levodopa outside the central nervous system. With the addition of a dopa-decarboxylase inhibitor, smaller doses of levodopa are effective.

a. **Sinemet®. Carbidopa** is combined with **levodopa** in **Sinemet®. Sinemet CR®,** a sustained release preparation, provides a controlled release of the drug into the gastrointestinal tract so that a dose of Sinemet is absorbed continuously over a longer period of time.

b. **Prolopa®/Benserazide®. Benserazide** is combined with levodopa in **Prolopa.**
(1) **Desired** and **undesirable effects** are identical to those for levodopa, alone. Many of the effects of levodopa are present but at a lower incidence and degree of severity.

(2) Dopamine replacement therapy is not completely effective, probably because it does not replicate, precisely, the physiology of the dopamine neuron that is impaired in Parkinson's disease.

4. **Amantadine hydrochloride (Symmetrel®),** developed as an antiviral agent, was discovered to be dopaminergic as well and has some use in Parkinson's disease. Amantadine stimulates the release of dopamine from the remaining intact dopaminergic neurons. It is useful as a primary drug in initiating therapy in patients with mild Parkinson's disease but is likely to be replaced by levodopa as time passes. Occasionally, patients with on-off effects who are taking maximum doses of levodopa can be given amantadine in conjunction with a slightly reduced dosage of levodopa.

   a. **Desired effects** are **decreased tremor, decreased rigidity, and increased facility of movement.**

   b. **Undesirable effects.** Initial drug therapy with amantadine produces the following side effects: **dry mouth, constipation, light-headedness, dizziness, weakness,** and occasional **orthostatic (postural) hypotension** (*see* Glossary). When added to levodopa, amantadine can produce the more severe side effects of **vivid dreams and nightmares, visual hallucinations, confusion, agitation,** and **overt psychosis.**

5. **Dopamine Receptor Agonists. Bromocriptine mesylate (Parlodel®)** and **pergolide mesylate (Permax®),** like levodopa, directly stimulate the dopamine receptor sites in the corpus striatum, thereby helping to offset the deficiency of dopamine responsible for the symptoms of Parkinson's disease. Unlike levodopa, usually these drugs are *not* used for initial primary therapy. Studies have compared levodopa and bromocriptine as initial therapy for Parkinson's disease. Results have revealed no difference, either in effectiveness or the incidence of immediate or late complications (for example, an on-off phenomenon).

   a. **Bromocriptine mesylate (Parlodel®)** may permit up to a 30% reduction of levodopa for patients who cannot tolerate the side effects of levodopa.
      (1) **Desired effect** is symptom relief when tolerance to levodopa develops or for on-off effects.
      (2) **Undesirable effects.** Common side effects are **gastrointestinal disturbance, postural hypotension,** and **fatigue.** Less common are **skin rash, headache, drowsiness, dizziness, syncope (fainting), nightmares, abnormal**

involuntary movements, depression, and **visual disturbances.** The common side effects of bromocriptine generally appear to be less troublesome than those associated with levodopa. Late side effects of **confusion** and **hallucinations** may take weeks to clear after the dose of bromocriptine is reduced. The **ankle edema** that occurs in some patients seems to clear rapidly when the drug is withdrawn. **Numbness** and **tingling** of the **fingers, muscle cramps,** and **gastrointestinal bleeding** may occur but are rare. **Drug induced changes in lung tissue** have been noted after long-term use of bromocriptine.

b. The mechanism of action of **pergolide mesylate (Permax®)** is similar to that of bromocriptine.

   (1) **Desired** and **undesirable effects** are similar to those of bromocriptine, although **cardiac arrhythmias** (*see* Glossary) are more likely to occur with pergolide.

c. **Combined therapy.** Some physicians are managing patients with a levodopa preparation initially and adding a low dose of a dopamine receptor agonist early in the course of the disease. Their goal is to decrease the incidence of on-off effects that occur later in the illness. However, to date, there has been no experimental study with data supporting a decision to combine the drugs.

6. **Monoamine Oxidase (MAO) Inhibitor. (Deprenyl®, Selegiline®, Eldepryl®). Deprenyl®** inhibits the enzyme that inactivates dopamine and slows the restorage of released dopamine at nerve terminals, thereby helping to correct the deficiency of dopamine thought to be responsible for the symptoms of Parkinson's disease. Possibly, **Deprenyl®** also slows the progression of Parkinson's disease.

Results of a trial of Deprenyl® in patients with newly diagnosed mild Parkinson's disease indicated that patients taking Deprenyl® did not progress to the point of requiring levodopa as quickly as did patients taking placebos. These results were confounded by the fact that Deprenyl® has a mild, therapeutic dopaminergic effect. There is still some controversy regarding the protective effect of Deprenyl®. Another study with a large number of subjects showed no difference in the progression of the disease with or without Deprenyl®.

a. **Desired effects** are mild relief of symptoms and slowed progression of the illness.

b. **Undesirable effects.** Mild side effects are **weakness, orthostatic hypotension, dry mouth,** and **insomnia.** More severe side effects are **dyskinesias, confusion, hallucinations, vivid dreams, depression, psychosis, aggravation of peptic ulcers,** and **gastrointestinal bleeding.** When Deprenyl is added to levodopa, the adverse effects of levodopa may develop or intensify. When this drug is taken with antihypertensive drugs, a significant decrease in blood pressure may occur.

7. Several drugs are under development and are not yet available for use in the United States. Table 2–2 contains a list of these drugs.

8. **Antipsychotic (neuroleptic) drugs.** When anti-Parkinson medications produce **psychiatric symptoms** (hallucinations, agitation, and psychosis) the best decision is to reduce the dosage of the drug. It is highly likely that at some point the Parkinsonian symptoms will increase. Traditional antipsychotics (*see* Schizophrenia) are dopamine receptor blockers and produce Parkinsonism. Recently, **Risperidone (Risperdal®) was developed.** This drug selectively blocks dopamine receptors. It does *not* block receptors in the basal ganglia in the area related to motor control.

a. **Desired effect** is relief of dopamine induced psychiatric symptoms without worsening of Parkinsonism.

Table 2–2. Anti-parkinson agents under development.

Anti-Parkinson Agent	Remarks
Cabergoline®	Synthetic dopamine agonist allowing less frequent dosing
Ropinirole®	Synthetic dopamine agonist with a chemical structure different from that of current agonist agents
Terguride®	Partial dopamine agonist; may prove useful in managing dyskinesias
Talipexole®	Dopamine agonist
Ro 40-7592®	Inhibits enzyme that metabolizes dopamine and crosses the blood-brain barrier.

b. Undesirable effects include **dizziness, hyperkinesia, somnolence,** and **nausea.** Some patients experience **Parkinsonism,** and, for these patients, the drug must be discontinued. Less common adverse reactions are **dry mouth, difficult urination, diarrhea, weight gain,** and **changes in sleep patterns and dreams.**

E. Effects of Anti-Parkinsonism Drugs on Communication

1. Even though dopamine replacement therapy may be successful in controlling other symptoms and signs of Parkinson's disease, speech and voice abnormalities seem to persist.

2. Dopamine agonists may produce **hallucinations,** usually **visual,** but, occasionally, **auditory. Paranoid thinking** has been reported as a side effect of levodopa. In addition, anti-Parkinson drugs can **impair concentration and memory,** and cause **confusion and disorientation.**

F. Alternatives to Pharmacologic Treatment

1. **Ablative Surgical Procedures. Pallidotomy** and **thalamotomy** have been used to decrease the symptoms of Parkinson's disease.

   a. Pallidotomy creates a small lesion in the globus pallidus and is performed to decrease bradykinesia. Balance and speech may improve even after a single, unilateral surgery.

   b. Thalamotomy creates a small lesion in the motor area of the thalamus and has been up to 98% effective in alleviating tremor. However, loss of muscle tone and impairment of balance and speech are associated risks and occur with greater frequency in bilateral surgeries.

2. **Tissue transplantation** into the striatum, the area of the basal ganglia that accepts dopamine from the substantia nigra, has been used with mixed results and remains controversial. Implantation of the tissue that produces dopamine is performed to increase the availability of dopamine.

   a. Adrenal Medulla Transplant. The adrenal medulla lies on top of the kidney. In the transplant procedure, a portion of the patient's own adrenal medulla is transplanted into the striatum to prevent the rejection by the immune system that could occur if an outside donor was used. It was hoped that the presence of these cells would increase the supply of available dopamine.

Unfortunately, the results were unsatisfactory, and **of the 300 or more patients who underwent adrenal medullary implantation in the United States in 1987 and 1988, only 19% demonstrated improvement after two years. Therefore, this procedure has been discontinued.**

b. **Fetal midbrain tissue** contains fetal cells that were destined to become substantia nigra. As in the case of adrenal medullary tissue, it is hoped that implantation of fetal membrane tissue will produce an increase in dopamine availability in the striatum. The reasoning underlying this method is that implanting dopamine-producing tissue from fetuses 6–10 weeks after conception will reinnervate the striatum, thereby establishing connections with the existing dopamine-receiving neurons.

(1) The first case of fetal implantation was performed in 1987, and the procedure continues to be improved.

(2) As many as eight or more fetal donors may be needed for maximum improvement of neurologic function in one patient with Parkinson's disease.

The MPTP Story

In the summer of 1982, in northern California, several patients experienced an inability to walk, move, and speak—the signs of severe Parkinson's disease. These patients had been street drug users of a synthetic chemical substance, a designer drug they had believed to be heroin. They were dubbed the "frozen addicts." It was discovered that the designer drug they ingested contained a contaminant, MPTP, that was metabolized in the brain to MPP+, a toxin that selectively destroyed the dopaminergic cells in the substantia nigra. Levodopa was administered to these patients, and, as in Parkinson's disease, the symptoms were relieved, significantly. However, the severe side effects of dyskinesia and hallucinations appeared.

MPTP was used to create the first animal model of Parkinson's disease. Experimenters at Yale University administered MPTP to monkeys and observed the same symptoms as demonstrated by the drug abusers. Next, they implanted monkey fetal tissue into the monkeys' brains and found that the symptoms disappeared. Finally,

(continued)

surgeons in Sweden, using human fetuses, performed a similar surgery on a patient from the northern California group. Subsequent to the surgery, that patient was able to decrease his dosage of levodopa by one-third and to maintain the dosage up to four years post-surgery.

In another experiment, it was discovered that administration of the MAO inhibitor, **Deprenyl**®, blocked the effect of **MPTP**. This supported the hypothesis that Parkinson's disease was the result of toxic exposure.

(3) The decision to implant fetal tissue is not an easy one. Even if implanted fetal cells survive and produce adequate dopamine, the input to these cells is not identical to input to the substantia nigra that occurs naturally. In addition, the use of fetal tissue has produced considerable controversy outside the area of medicine.

3. **Speech-Voice Therapy.** Until recently, there was little to indicate the efficacy of speech therapy for the dysarthria of Parkinson's disease. Procedures emphasizing articulation therapy; rate control; and other methods for improving prosody; and counseling in the use of pragmatic functions resulted in little carry-over from the clinic into the patient's natural environment.

a. **Isometric exercises** to achieve vocal fold closure and emphasizing **increasing, calibrating,** and **maintaining voice volume** (loudness), have improved overall speech intelligibility as a byproduct of the increase in vocal loudness.

G. RECOMMENDED READINGS

Bayles, K. A., & Kaszniak, A.W. (1987). *Communication and cognition in normal aging.* Boston: Little, Brown.

Cummings, J. L. (1992). Depression and Parkinson's disease: A review. *American Journal of Psychiatry. 149,* 443–454.

Darley, F. L., Aronson, A. E., & Brown, J. R. (1975). *Motor speech disorders.* Philadelphia: W.B. Saunders.

Goetz, C. G., DeLong, M. R., Penn, R. D., & Bakay, R. A. E. (1993). Neurosurgical horizons in Parkinson's disease. *Neurology, 43,* 1–7.

Long, J. W. (1992). *The essential guide to prescription drugs.* New York: Harper-Collins.

Ramig, L. O. (1990, January). *Changes in phonation of Parkinson's disease patients following voice therapy.* Paper presented to the Clinical Dysarthria Conference, San Antonio, TX.

Sacks, O. (1983). *Awakenings.* New York: E. P. Dutton.

Sherman, D. (1988). Neurologic diseases. In Stein, J. F. (Ed.), *Internal medicine: Diagnosis and therapy.* Boston/Toronto: Little, Brown.

II. ADDITIONAL CONDITIONS PRODUCING PARKINSONISM

A. Although the symptoms and signs of most Parkinsonian conditions are similar to those of Parkinson's disease, the two conditions are clinically distinguishable. The patient presents with Parkinsonian and additional neurological symptoms, as well. These symptoms can include **impaired ocular movements, spinocerebellar, corticospinal and autonomic motor neuron degeneration; peripheral neuropathy;** and **dementia.**

1. **Post-encephalitic Parkinsonism**

   a. **General features, symptoms, and signs**
      (1) The symptoms and signs of post-encephalitic parkinsonism are similar to those of Parkinson's disease, but the former usually involves more autonomic dysfunction. Some additional symptoms are **blepharospasm (frequent and tight closing of the eyelids),** and **oculogyric crisis in which patients experience forced deviation of the eyes, upward.**

   b. **Features, symptoms, and signs of communication impairment** are similar to those of Parkinson's disease.

   c. **Pharmacologic treatment.** See Levodopa.

   d. **Effects of the drugs on communication.** *See* Table 2–1.

   e. **Alternative treatments** will vary with the severity of the communication disorder.

2. **Progressive Supranuclear Palsy (PSP); Steele-Richardson-Olszewski Syndrome**

   a. **Definition/Cause.** Histologically, neuronal cell loss, gliosis, and neurofibrillary tangles are present in the brain stem, basal ganglia, and cerebellar nuclei. Usually, there is marked atrophy of the midbrain and pons.

b. General features, symptoms, and signs

    (1) The failure of conjugate gaze (supranuclear ophthalmoplegia) is a prominent feature. Disturbed eye motility is manifested, initially, by loss of downward and upward gaze. Later, all eye movements are affected, and, eventually, patients lose all ability to move their eyes.

    (2) Additional symptoms and signs are dystonic rigidity of the neck and upper trunk, pseudobulbar palsy, and a tendency to fall backward. Often, the rigidity is extensor rather than flexor. Therefore, posture is less forward and stooped than in Parkinson's disease.

    (3) Parkinsonian manifestations such as **bradykinesia, masked facies,** and **poor postural reflexes** are observed. Usually, tremor is minimal or is not present at all.

c. Features, symptoms, and signs of communication impairment

    (1) A mixed—hypokinetic, spastic, and ataxic—dysarthria is compatible with the neurologic findings of PSP. The two prominent components of the dysarthria are hypokinesia and spasticity. Ataxia is the least prominent component. Speech is slow and hypophonic. Eventually, the patient may become mute.

    (2) **Palilalia** and sound intrusions resembling throat clearing, tongue clicking, and other extraneous noises may be observed.

    (3) **Language** usually is normal, although a decrease in the use of gestures occurs, probably because of the associated bradykinesia. Dementia with memory loss is a salient feature of the impaired cognition associated with the later stages of the disease.

d. Pharmacologic treatment

    (1) **Levodopa** has much less effect on the symptoms of PSP than on the symptoms of Parkinson's disease. The drug may be effective, temporarily, for some patients with PSP.

       (i) **Desired effect.** Decrease of symptoms.

       (ii) **Undesirable effects. Dry mouth, blurred vision, gastrointestinal disturbance, cardiac arrhythmias, postural hypotension,** and **syncope** are reported side effects. For a complete list of side effects of levodopa *see* Table 2–1.

(2) Occasionally, **bromocriptine** is used in an attempt to reduce symptoms. Common side effects of bromocriptine are **fatigue, lethargy,** and **orthostatic hypotension.** For a discussion of undesirable effects of **bromocriptine,** *see* Parkinson's disease.

e. **Effects of the drugs on communication** are similar to the effects of the drugs on Parkinson's disease.

f. **Alternatives to pharmacologic treatment**
   (1) Speech therapy. The success of therapy for dysarthria of PSP is questionable, particularly in patients who experience memory loss and dementia. Counseling of caregivers regarding methods for achieving optimum communication may be beneficial.

3. **Multiple system disease**

   a. **Definition/causes and symptoms**
   Major subgroups of multiple system disease have been identified: The first has predominant cerebellar features (olivopontocerebellar degeneration). The second has predominant autonomic features such as orthostatic hypotension (a drop in blood pressure on assuming an upright posture without associated rise in pulse), as in Shy-Drager syndrome. Additional causes of parkinsonism are striatonigral degeneration; poisons such as carbon monoxide, cyanide, and manganese; and drug ingestion.

   b. Pharmacologic treatments are similar to those for Parkinson's disease but may not be effective. The symptom of postural hypotension in Shy-Drager syndrome may be reduced with **9-fluorocortisone (Florinef®).**

B. Recommended Readings

Metter, E. J., & Hanson, W. R. (1991). Dysarthria in progressive supranuclear palsy. In C. A. Moore, K. M. Yorkston, & D. R. Beukelman, (Eds.), *Dysarthria and apraxia of speech: Perspectives on management.* Baltimore: Paul H. Brookes.

III. MYASTHENIA GRAVIS

A. Definition/Cause

1. Myasthenia gravis is an **autoimmune disease** in which the immune system produces antibodies in the blood that impair the transmission of nerve impulses to muscle. There is a disturbance at the synapse between the nerve and the muscle, that is, the neuromuscular junction. The neurotransmitter involved is acetylcholine (Ach).

2. The mechanisms responsible for formation of the destructive antibodies leading to myasthenia gravis are not well understood. There is no pattern of heredity that predicts its development as in other diseases (see Huntington's disease). There is, however, a genetic factor that produces susceptibility to autoimmune diseases in families; and individuals with first degree relatives with autoimmune disorders are at increased risk to develop autoimmune disorders. Furthermore, individuals with one autoimmune disorder have an increased probability of developing additional autoimmune disorders.

3. The majority of women with myasthenia develop it as young adults, while the majority of men with the disease develop it later in life. The peak incidence is 50–59 years of age.

B. General Features, Symptoms, and Signs

1. Physiologically, myasthenia produces fatigue of muscles. Patients complain of weakness that increases with the duration of activity.

   a. Early in the disease, symptoms may occur only in late afternoon or evening. Symptoms may fluctuate from minute to minute, hour to hour, or day to day. In some patients, the disease progresses, and symptoms become continuous.

   b. Spontaneous remissions can occur but usually are temporary and occur early in the disease. Other illness may precipitate an exacerbation.

2. **Ptosis (drooping of the eyelid)** and **diplopia (double vision)** are common. Up to 80% of patients present initially with these symptoms. For about 15% of patients, there is never progression to involve other muscles. These patients are said to have **ocular myasthenia.**

3. Other patients develop symptoms in muscles other than the eyes. Weakness of bulbar muscles causing dysarthria and dysphagia is frequent. The remainder of the patients have generalized involvement of eyes, bulbar muscles, and extremity muscles.

4. In 65% of young patients there may be a **persistent, enlarged thymus gland.** About 10% of patients, usually, older men, have a **thymoma,** a tumor that is usually benign but may be locally invasive.

C. Features, Symptoms, and Signs of Communication Impairment

These patients display a **flaccid dysarthria.** This speech contains the following features: at the beginning of an utterance, speech usually is intelligible, but as the patient continues speaking, fatigue of speech musculature becomes evident as hypernasality, deterioration of articulation, onset and increase of dysphonia, and reduction of loudness are observed. Intelligibility deteriorates until the speech becomes impossible to understand.

D. Pharmacologic Treatment

1. **Edrophonim chloride (Tensilon®)** is used to confirm the diagnosis of myasthenia. It is administered intravenously, as the patient is observed for improvement of speech and other behavioral signs. The drug is short acting—2–20 minutes, and its influence is reversible. If speech and other behaviors improve during the drug effect, the diagnosis of myasthenia gravis is confirmed.

   a. **Desired effect** is diagnosis of myasthenia gravis.

   b. **Undesirable effects** are excessive **sweating, tearing, salivation,** and **gastrointestinal disturbance.** Occasionally, **cardiac arrhythmias** have been precipitated by Tensilon® testing.

2. Drugs used to treat myasthenia are designed either to enhance the action of Ach by inhibiting acetylcholinesterase or by using immunosuppressant drugs, suppressing the immune response that is producing the antibodies.

   a. **Acetylcholinesterase inhibitors. Pyridostigmine (Mestinon®),** the most commonly used drug, inhibits cholinesterase, the enzyme that destroys Ach.
      (1) **Desired effect is an increased level of Ach** that facilitates the stimulation of muscular activity that leads to decreased weakness.

(2) **Undesirable effects. Diarrhea, excessive salivation,** and **gastrointestinal disturbance** are the most common side effects of Mestinon. Less common side effects are **skin rash, nervousness,** and **confusion.** An excess of acetylcholinesterase medication may produce **weakness,** and signs of too much may not be distinguishable from signs of too little medication. Usually, this is a problem only for patients with severe myasthenia who are receiving high doses of medication for maximum effect.

b. **Neostigmine (Prostigmin®)** is an acetylcholinesterase inhibitor with desired and undesirable effects similar to those of pyridostigmine.

c. **Corticosteroids** Many patients whose symptoms cannot be controlled adequately with acetylcholinesterase inhibitors may require immunosuppressants. **Corticosteroids** are the mainstay of immunosuppressant therapy in myasthenia gravis. **Prednisone® and Dexamethasone®** suppress the immune response producing the antibodies that cause the illness, and have similar desired and undesirable effects. Approaches to the use of steroids vary. A small dose that is gradually increased until symptoms are controlled can be followed by a gradual decrease to a dose with continued symptom control. Alternatively, treatment can be initiated with a large dose and gradually tapered to the lowest dosage demonstrated to control the symptoms. Sometimes this approach produces a temporary increase in weakness and requires hospitalization.

(1) **Desired effect is a decrease in weakness,** occurring within a few weeks if drug therapy is initiated with low doses that are increased. Large doses of the drug should produce decreased weakness within a shorter period of time.

(2) **Undesirable effects.** Although short-term use of Prednisone® (up to 10 days) usually is well tolerated, long-term use (exceeding two weeks) is associated with many possible adverse effects. The incidence and severity of these side effects increase with the duration of therapy. *See* Table 2–3 for the effects of short- and long-term use of Prednisone®.

> Prednisone® is withdrawn gradually and never should be discontinued abruptly. Approximately 90% of patients remain dependent upon long-term use for maintaining improvement, and only about 10% are able to withdraw successfully and remain in remission.

Table 2–3. Effects of short and long term use of prednisone

Short-term Use	Long-term Use
Skin rash, headache, dizziness, insomnia, indigestion, muscle cramping and weakness, and growth of facial hair	Altered mood and personality, cataracts, glaucoma, hypertension, susceptibility to infections, susceptibility to peptic ulcer disease, susceptibility to pulmonary embolism, Cushing's syndrome, and thinning and fragility of the skin

   d. Dexamethasone (Decadron®) often is used if treatment with Prednisone fails to control the symptoms of myasthenia.

     (1) Desired effect is improvement in function or **remission of symptoms** occurring in most cases and continuing for 3 months or longer after the drug is discontinued.

     (2) Undesirable effects are **increased appetite, weight gain, retention of salt and water, excretion of potassium** and **increased susceptibility to infection. Cushing's syndrome** (*see* Glossary) and other common adverse effects of corticosteroids are possible side effects.

   e. Azathioprene (Imuran®) is an immunosuppressant that is less toxic when used over time than moderate or high doses of long-term corticosteroids. Imuran may be used alone or to reduce the steroid requirement. However, if used in excessive doses, Imuran has a higher potential for morbidity than do steroid drugs. Therefore, Imuran may not be prescribed until patients have shown an inability to tolerate low doses of corticosteroids.

     (1) Desired effect. Improved function usually requires months, often up to a year to develop. Continued drug therapy may be required for 12–36 months. A high dose of Imuran® may be needed to maintain improvement.

     (2) Undesirable effects. Mild side effects of Imuran are **skin rash, loss of appetite, gastrointestinal disturbance,** and **sores on the lip or in the mouth.** More serious side effects are **joint and muscle pain, pancreatitis** (*see* Glossary), **bone marrow depression** with **increased susceptibility** to **infection, liver damage,** and **drug induced pneumonia.** There may be an increased risk of **subsequent lymphoma and leukemia.**

f. **Cyclophosphamide (Cytoxan®)** may be prescribed for patients who cannot be weaned off or to a small dose of steroids. It may be used under the same conditions as Imuran.

    (1) **Desired effect** is reduction of the steroid requirement.

    (2) **Undesirable effects** are **headache, dizziness, loss of scalp hair,** and **loss of appetite.** More adverse reactions are **bone marrow depression with increased susceptibility to infection, liver damage with jaundice, kidney damage,** and **drug-induced damage of heart and lung tissue.** A few patients develop a **hemorrhagic cystitis (bleeding from irritation of the bladder)** that may be severe, or even fatal. There may be an increased **risk of lymphoma and leukemia.**

    (3) Cytoxan® and Imuran® share many features, but Imuran is considered to be a slightly more benign drug with fewer dangerous side effects.

g. **Cyclosporin (Sandimmune®)**

    (1) **Desired effect** is control of symptoms and reduction of the steroid requirement.

    (2) **Undesirable effects** include **hypertension, tremor, hirsutism (growth of hair), hypertrophy of gums,** and **gastrointestinal disorders.** The most significant adverse effect is **kidney damage,** and therefore, renal function must be monitored carefully.

    (3) Cyclosporin has less effect on the bone marrow than does other drugs.

    (4) Although there are limited outcome data regarding the efficacy of using Cyclosporin to treat myasthenia or other neurological disease, its use for treatment of these diseases is increasing.

E. Effects of the Drugs on Communication

1. Pharmacologic treatment improves strength and endurance of bulbar musculature, thereby **decreasing dysarthria,** and **improving the intelligibility of speech.**

2. Corticosteroids can cause **confusion, disorientation,** and **impaired concentration and memory** as side effects of long-term use.

F. Alternatives to Pharmacologic Treatment

1. **Thymectomy**. Removal of a thymoma often results in improved function. For patients with generalized myasthenia, exploration of

the mediastinum to remove remnants of thymic tissue, or any visible thymus gland, generally is recommended. Thymectomy may provide a cure, improve function, or allow a lower dosage of drugs to control symptoms of myasthenia.

2. **Plasmapheresis**. During plasmapheresis, the patient's blood is removed and the plasma exchanged for appropriate substitute fluids, thus eliminating the destructive circulating antibodies and providing relief from symptoms. Because this procedure does not stop the ongoing production of the antibodies, symptoms tend to return within a few weeks unless additional drug therapy is undertaken. Simultaneous initiation of immunosuppressant drug therapy usually is part of the overall therapeutic plan. Because of its almost immediate effect, **plasmapheresis** is useful when preparing a patient for thymectomy or during severe symptomatic periods that require hospitalization.

3. **Speech/Voice Therapy** may be indicated to decrease the dysarthria and improve the intelligibility of speech.

F. Recommended Readings

Long, J. W. (1992). *The essential guide to prescription drugs*. New York: Harper-Collins.
Walshe, T. M. (1991). Diseases of the nerve and muscle. In M. A. Samuels, (Ed.) *Manual of neurology. Diagnosis and therapy* (4th ed., pp. 335–370). Boston/Toronto. Little, Brown.

IV. AMYOTROPHIC LATERAL SCLEROSIS (ALS)

A. Definition/Cause

1. ALS is a **progressive, degenerative,** and **fatal disease** involving motor neurons of the cortex, brainstem, and spinal cord. As the disease progresses, there is degeneration of both the upper and lower motor neuron systems. Presently the etiology is unknown, but in Guam, where there is a very high incidence of ALS, Parkinson's disease, and dementia occurring in combination, it is thought that chronic exposure to a plant toxin with neuroexcitatory activity may be associated with the development of the disease.

2. One **hypothesis concerning the cause** of ALS is that glutamate, the primary excitatory neurotransmitter in the CNS, accumulates to a toxic level at synapses. This causes neurons to die.

3. The mean age of onset is 56 years. There are twice as many men as women with ALS. In 50% of cases, death occurs within three years after identification of symptoms. Approximately 10% of patients survive up to 10 years, and some patients live as long as 20 years after diagnosis.

B. General Features, Symptoms, and Signs

The most common presenting symptom is weakness of the upper and lower extremities. Weakness of bulbar muscles resulting in dysarthria and dysphagia is common.

C. Features, Symptoms, and Signs of Communication Impairment

The combined upper and lower motor neuron involvement results in a mixed, spastic-flaccid dysarthria with severely compromised speech intelligibility. Imprecise consonants, hypernasality, slow rate, and harsh voice quality are prominent features of the dysarthria of ALS.

D. Pharmacologic Treatment

1. Drug treatment for ALS has been disappointing. No drug has been shown to cure the disease, and control of symptoms is problematic. The therapeutic effects of the drugs are overcome by the progression of the disease.

   a. **Thyrotropin Releasing Hormone (TRH).** TRH stimulates the release of thyrotropin from the anterior pituitary and increases activity of the thyroid gland. In the early 1980s, it was found that neurons in the spinal cord contained receptors for TRH, although the purpose of these receptors was unclear. One hypothesis was that TRH had a "tropic effect on neurons" and its presence was necessary to maintain the health of the neurons. Further, it was hypothesized that if endogenous TRH is deficient in ALS, then exogenous TRH can replace the deficit. This theory led to trials of therapy with TRH. Unfortunately, early success in decreasing or eliminating symptoms was tempered by the lack of sustained benefit. Also, the need for parenteral rather than oral administration, with high cost, hyperthyroidism, and other substantial side effects, were factors that argued against the use of the drug. Currently, TRH is rarely, if ever, used to treat ALS.

b. **Riluzole.** Results of a recent study of **riluzole**, an agent thought to modulate the neurotransmitter glutamate, indicated that after 12 months, 74% of patients (N = 155) in a riluzole group were still alive compared to 57% of patients in a placebo group. Moreover, the deterioration of muscle strength was significantly slower in the experimental versus the control group. Adverse side effects of riluzole included asthenia (*see* Glossary), **spasticity, mild elevations in aminotransferase levels**, and a **mild to moderate increase in blood pressure**. The investigators reported that the drug seemed to delay crippling symptoms and death and that it "slowed the curve of the disease." They agreed that additional studies with a larger number of ALS patients are needed to draw definitive conclusions, and suggested that decisions to prescribe riluzole should be deferred until further clinical trials are conducted.

c. **Gabapentin (Neurontin®) and Lamotrigine (Lamictal®)** are new anticonvulsants (*see* Epilepsy) that may be prescribed for patients with ALS. Gabapentin acts like GABA, the primary inhibitory neurotransmitter in the central nervous system and may counteract the neurotransmitters glutamate and aspartate. Lamotrigine inhibits the release of glutamate and aspartate (*see* Chapter 1). For further discussion regarding Gabapentin and Lamotrigine, *see* Anticonvulsants.

2. **Treatment of symptoms: Spasticity**. (*see* Multiple Sclerosis for a description of spasticity). A variety of agents have been used to treat spasticity. **Baclofen (Lioresal®), diazepam (Valium®), and dantrolene (Dantrium®)** are the three most frequently used drugs.

a. **Baclofen (Lioresal®)** is the drug of choice for the treatment of spasticity.
   (1) **Desired effect** is reduction of painful flexor and extensor spasms, without producing increased weakness.
   (2) **Undesirable effect** is **drowsiness**, that may diminish with continued use. Occasionally, **more persistent drowsiness** and **unsteadiness** occur. The **loss of ability to bear weight** is experienced by some patients who are very weak. Baclofen can cause **elevation in liver function tests** in some patients. This may reverse when the dose is lowered or may require that the drug be discontinued.

    b. Diazepam (Valium®)
      (1) Desired effect is reduction of spasticity.
      (2) Undesirable effects. The mild side effects of **drowsiness, fatigue,** and **unsteadiness** are common and may be temporary. More serious side effects are **skin rash, dizziness, fainting, blurred vision, diplopia, dysarthria, sweating,** and **nausea.** Liver damage with impaired production of white blood cells, fever, and pharyngitis has been observed.

      Diazepam can impair mental alertness, judgment, physical coordination, and **reaction time.** Alcohol may increase the absorption of diazepam and add to its depressant effects.

    c. Dantrolene (Dantrium®)
      (1) Desired effect. Dantrolene may be prescribed for severe spasticity when baclofen and diazepam are not effective. It is most useful in patients with very little remaining function but marked spasticity that is interfering with nursing care.
      (2) Undesirable effects. Dantrolene *always* causes **decoupling of excitation-contraction in muscle.** Therefore, the drug always produces increased weakness. Additional side effects are **drowsiness, dizziness,** and **diarrhea.** A dose-related hepatotoxic reaction can be fatal (*see* Glossary). Low dosages are not likely to cause this reaction.

  3. Treatment of symptoms: Flaccid Weakness. No medications are available that improve strength due to loss of the motor neurons that connect with the muscles.

E. Effects of the Drugs on Communication

  1. TRH seemed to produce early success in controlling dysarthria. In one case study of a patient with severe dysarthria, it was reported that although the patient's speech became more intelligible, factors that contraindicated the use of the drug made it necessary to withdraw it. After a period of less than three months after withdrawal, the benefits disappeared, and the severe dysarthria returned.

  2. The effects of **riluzole** on communication are unknown at this time.

F. Alternatives to Pharmacologic Treatment

  1. Surgical interventions involving **nasopharyngeal muscle augmentation** and **pharyngeal flap** have been tried.

2. Patients who are not able to obtain sufficient velopharyngeal closure for intelligible speech may benefit from a **palatal lift prosthesis**.

3. **Speech therapy** to improve velopharyngeal valving competency may be attempted.

4. **Augmentative communication devices** will be needed as the disease progresses and the severity of the dysarthria increases.

5. **Counseling** the patient and caregiver is essential throughout the course of the disease to suggest the most effective methods for achieving optimum communication.

6. **Physical therapy** may help to minimize atrophy and prevent contractures. Although attempts to "build up" muscles have not been successful, preserving strength for accomplishing activities of daily living is an essential component of physical therapy for the patient with ALS.

7. **Motorized and mechanical appliances** such as wheelchairs, lifts, and hospital beds can help the patient to obtain maximum independence.

G. Recommended Readings

Bensimon, G., Lacombliz, V., Meininger, V., & the ALS/Riluzole Study Group. (1994). A controlled trial of riluzole in amyotrophic lateral sclerosis. *New England Journal of Medicine, 330*(9), 585–591.

Vogel, D. (1989). Effects of thyrotropin-releasing hormone on dysarthria in amyotrophic lateral sclerosis. In K. M. Yorkston & D. R. Beukelman (Eds.), *Recent advances in clinical dysarthria* (pp. 109–116). Austin, TX: Pro-Ed.

Walshe, T. M. (1991). Diseases of the nerve and muscle. In M. A. Samuels, (Ed.), *Manual of neurology. Diagnosis and therapy* (pp. 335–370). Boston/Toronto: Little, Brown.

V. MULTIPLE SCLEROSIS (MS)

A. Definition/Cause

1. **MS** is characterized by loss of myelin and preservation of axons. The diagnosis of MS is based on the history of a fluctuating course with exacerbations and remissions. Five to 10% of patients develop a more chronic, progressive illness. Most often, these are men. Usually, the spinal cord is the site of the predominant involvement.

   a. Typically **MRI** shows diffuse and progressive demyelination in the white matter adjacent to the ventricles, the optic nerves, brainstem, cerebellum, and spinal cord.

    b. Cerebrospinal fluid (CSF) studies may show inflammation, abnormal immunoglobulin production in the CNS, or myelin breakdown products—myelin basic protein.

    c. Onset of symptoms usually occurs between the ages of 15–50 years, although cases outside this age range have been reported.

    d. The actual **cause** of multiple sclerosis **is unknown**, although there are statistical clues. About 60% of patients with MS share the genetic tissue type DR2, and first degree relatives are at higher risk for developing the disease. Sixty percent are female. The incidence is twice as high in individuals who grew up in temperate, rather than subtropical, latitudes.

    e. MS is an **autoimmune disease** in which part of the body's defense system turns against normal cells. In patients with MS, the immediate target of this self-destruction is **myelin**—the protective covering that electrically insulates nerve fibers in the central nervous system. Usually, the attack on myelin is led by helper T cells that destroy what the cells assume to be an invader.

B. General Features, Symptoms, and Signs

    1. Early in the disease, when abnormalities detected by neurologic examination are minimal, and before more common symptoms appear, patients may be diagnosed as **hysterical** or **depressed**.

    2. Sensory complaints (parathesias, numbness); **visual problems** (unilateral or bilateral visual loss, diplopia); motor abnormalities (paralysis, clumsiness, unsteadiness, loss of balance) and **vestibular** and **cerebellar** symptoms (vertigo, dizziness, disequilibrium) are common.

    3. Over one-half of patients experience at least one attack of **optic neuritis**, an abrupt (usually over 2–3 days) loss of vision resulting from optic nerve demyelination. Most undergo substantial recovery in subsequent weeks.

    4. Motor abnormalities (spastic weakness) may be identified by the presence of hyperactive deep tendon reflexes including positive Babinski signs (upgoing great toe on stimulation of the sole of the foot).

        a. Spasticity is defined as increased resistance of a joint and its muscles to passive movement. It is a loss of the fine control between incoming proprioceptive sensory input from the joints/muscles and outgoing motor impulses that maintain the muscle at a length and tension appropriate for the joint position and ongoing activities. With loss of input from descending pathways, the reflex muscle contraction stimulated by joint movement is disinhibited and produces an increase in muscle tone. Mild spasticity may be manifested as a simple loss of fine motor control, while more pronounced and prolonged spasticity results in a jerkiness in response to movements and contractures of the joints.

5. Many patients with MS experience cerebellar intention tremor or ataxia at some time during the illness. Table 2–4 lists symptoms and signs of multiple sclerosis.

C. Features, Symptoms, and Signs of Communication Impairment

1. A **mixed flaccid, spastic**, and/or **ataxic dysarthria** with mild to grossly defective articulation frequently is observed. Slow, laborious speech rate, severe disruption of prosody; marked hypernasality, and severe, harsh, strained-strangled phonation have been noted. Impaired control of loudness, excessive and equal or reduced stress, and monopitch are additional characteristics. The type and severity of the dysarthria are directly related to the extent of the neurologic involvement.

2. **Cognitive impairment** has been identified in a subset of patients.

D. Pharmacologic Treatment

1. Presently, there is no drug that will cure MS. Drug therapy may be focused on reducing the number of attacks of demyelination or on

Table 2–4. Symptoms and signs of multiple sclerosis.

Sensory complaints

Optic neuritis

Spasticity and motor abnormalities

Cerebellar disorders

Dysarthria and dysphagia

Bladder, bowel, and sexual dysfunction

Mood disorders

Shooting/lancinating pains of pelvic girdle, shoulder, and face reducing the damage caused by individual attacks. With the large majority of attacks (exacerbations), patients undergo substantial recovery with no drug therapy. Therefore, it is difficult to determine the efficacy of drug therapy on recovery from the attacks of multiple sclerosis.

2. Several drugs have been identified that may reduce the duration of acute exacerbations. Powerful immunosuppressants are used in patients with severe, disabling chronic progressive MS, but it has been difficult to demonstrate a substantial benefit of using these drugs. The following sections are discussions of immunosuppressant drugs used for treatment of MS.

a. **Adrenocorticotrophic hormone** (ACTH) stimulates the production of adrenal corticosteroids by the patient's own adrenal glands. The original placebo-controlled drug outcome study utilized ACTH. Results of this study showed no difference in the degree of residual deficit between patients on ACTH and patients taking placebos. However, patients did recover a little sooner while taking ACTH, and for a period of time neurologists prescribed the drug for patients who experienced attacks of MS. ACTH must be administered intravenously which requires hospitalization. Therefore, in time, physicians preferred to prescribe corticosteroids, an oral medication.

(1) **Desired effect** is the reduction of symptoms of acute exacerbation.

(2) **Undesirable effects** are **fluid retention** possibly resulting in **hypertension, gastric irritation** possibly resulting in **hemorrhage,** and **restlessness, anxiety, insomnia, infection,** and **sepsis**.

b. **Corticosteroids** can be administered orally, are less expensive, and may be as effective as ACTH in reducing the duration of acute exacerbations of MS. These drugs are used by many physicians to treat attacks of demyelination and optic neuritis. Corticosteroids commonly prescribed for patients with MS are **Prednisone®, Dexamethasone (Decadron®),** and oral preparations of methylprednisolone (Medrol®). Desired and undesirable effects are similar for these drugs.

(1) **Desired effects**. Shortening the duration of acute attacks.

(2) **Undesirable effects**. Complications and adverse reactions to corticosteroid therapy are time and dose related. **Alterations of mood,** and **fluid retention and weight gain** are the primary adverse effects of short-term use. Long-term corticosteroid therapy is avoided whenever pos-

sible. An undesirable effect of chronic steroid use is **Cushing's syndrome** (*see* Glossary). See Table 2–3 for a list of side effects of long and short-term use of corticosteroids.

c. **Azathioprine (Imuran®)** is an immunosuppressant that is less toxic in long-term use than high or moderate doses of corticosteroids. Imuran® may be used alone or in combination with steroids. For desired and undesirable effects of Imuran, see Myasthenia Gravis.

d. **Cyclophosphamide (Cytoxan®)** is an immunosuppressant that is somewhat more powerful and more toxic than Imuran® Cytoxan® may be used alone or in combination with steroids.
   (1) **Desired effect** is to arrest the progression of the disease and to limit the number and severity of neurological deficits.
   (2) **Undesirable effects**. Mild side effects are **headache, dizziness, loss of scalp hair,** and **loss of appetite**. More adverse reactions are **bone marrow depression with increased susceptibility to infection, liver damage with jaundice,** and **drug-induced damage of heart and lung tissue**. A few patients develop a **hemorrhagic cystitis** (bleeding from irritation of the bladder) which may be severe or fatal. There may be an increased **risk of lymphoma** and **leukemia**.

   Cyclophosphamide and Imuran® share many features, but most physicians consider Imuran® to be the slightly more benign drug.

e. Results of a recent clinical study involving a large sample (372) of MS patients, revealed that patients receiving high doses of **beta interferon (Betaseron®)** experienced one third fewer episodes of exacerbation than those given a placebo. After several years, the area of the brain in which lesions appeared decreased by 4.2% in patients taking high doses of beta interferon, while those given a placebo showed a 19.4% increase. It was unfortunate that even when there were no symptoms, patients continued to develop active lesions as observed on serial MRI scans. This finding convinced some physicians to treat all MS patients with beta interferon, even if the patient experienced only occasional exacerbations at very long intervals.
   (1) Beta interferon must be administered by injection for a number of years until the patient has had no exacerbations for a long period of time and has reached an age when the MS has become quiescent (approximately 40–50 years of age).

(i) **Desired effect** is to decrease or eliminate new demyelinating events and exacerbations of symptoms.

(ii) **Undesirable effects** include **local inflammation** at the site of injections and a **flu-like syndrome**.

> When Betaseron® first became available, there was not enough of it to supply all the patients for whom the drug was appropriate. The manufacturer solicited the names of patients from neurologists in the United States and performed a lottery to select the patients who would receive the medication.

f. **Coplyner** (Cop 1) has been used to modulate the body's spontaneous immunologic reactions to myelin and decrease the occurrence of exacerbations in MS. Although side effects are mild **(flushing, palpations, muscle tightness, difficulty breathing,** and **anxiety)**, Cop 1 cannot be taken orally and must be administered by subcutaneous injection twice a day.

g. In a recent trial of 30 patients with relapsing-remitting early stage MS, half of the patients were given daily capsules of **bovine myelin**. The other half received a placebo. During the year-long study, 23 placebo-control subjects suffered exacerbations of their MS compared with only six myelin-treated patients. Although 6 of the treated patients improved significantly over the year, improvement was observed for only 2 of the placebo-control subjects. Moreover, no side effects or infections were observed for the treated patients. The investigators cautioned that this is by no means a proven method for curing MS, but they see this as a possible method for turning off the immune responses with an oral drug.

2. Treatment of symptoms: Spasticity

A variety of agents have been used to treat **spasticity**. The following are three used most frequently:

a. **Baclofen (Lioresal®)** has emerged as the drug of choice for treatment of spasticity.

(1) **Desired effect** is reduction of painful flexor and extensor spasms without producing increased weakness.

(2) **Undesirable effects** include **drowsiness**, that may diminish with continued use. Occasionally, more **persistent**

drowsiness and **unsteadiness** occur. The loss of ability to bear weight is experienced by some patients who are very weak. **Baclofen** can cause **elevation in liver function tests** in some patients. This may reverse when the dose is lowered or may require that the drug be discontinued. More serious side effects include **liver damage with jaundice** and **abnormally low blood counts**.

b. **Diazepam (Valium®)**
   (1) **Desired effect** is reduction of spasticity.
   (2) **Undesirable effects**. The mild side effects of **drowsiness, fatigue,** and **unsteadiness** are common and may be temporary. More serious side effects are **skin rash, dizziness, fainting, blurred vision, diplopia, dysarthria, sweating, and nausea. Liver damage with jaundice and an abnormally low blood platelet count** have been reported. **Bone marrow depression with impaired production of white blood cells, fever,** and **pharyngitis** has been observed.

> **Diazepam can impair mental alertness, judgment, physical coordination,** and **reaction time**. Alcohol may increase the absorption of diazepam and add to its depressant effects.

c. **Dantrolene (Dantrium®)**
   (1) **Desired effect**. Dantrolene may be prescribed for severe spasticity when Baclofen and Diazepam are not effective. It is most useful in patients with very little remaining function and marked spasticity that is interfering with nursing care.
   (2) **Undesirable effects**. Dantrolene **always** causes **decoupling of excitation-contraction in muscle.** Therefore, the drug **always** produces **increased weakness**. Additional side effects are **drowsiness, dizziness,** and **diarrhea**. Although a dose-related **hepatotoxic reaction** (*see* Glossary) can be fatal, low dosages are not likely to cause this reaction.

3. Drug therapy for **cerebellar dysfunction** is disappointing. Drugs that have been tried are **5-hydroxytryptophan** and **isoniazid (INH)**. These drugs may decrease postural instability and dysarthria. Some physicians have reported INH to be effective, but others have been unable to confirm any benefit. In addition, INH is associated with a **high incidence of hepatotoxicity**.

E. Effects of the Drugs on Communication

1. **Depression, emotional lability, psychosis**, and the communication deficits associated with them may be related to the drug therapy or may be a consequence of the disease. *See* Psychiatric Disorders for discussions of depression and schizophrenia. Treatment with antidepressants may be effective for treating the complications of MS.

2. The drugs designed to shorten the exacerbation and lengthen the remission periods may also decrease the severe dysarthria.

F. Alternatives to Pharmacologic Treatment

1. **Physical Therapy.** For treatment of tremor and ataxia, weighting of the affected limbs and general conditioning techniques may be beneficial. **Physical therapy** can be useful for treating weakness due to lack of muscle use or for maintaining range of motion and assisting in gait training.

2. **Thalamotomy** may be of benefit for a small, selected group of patients with chronic, disabling tremors.

3. **Psychotherapy** is recommended for treating reactive depression.

4. **Speech and Voice Therapy.** Techniques for controlling vocal loudness and harshness often are beneficial, as is therapy for articulation impairment. A "top-down" approach to treatment of dysarthric speech, emphasizing pragmatics of communication, may be helpful. Different exacerbations may produce different dysarthric symptoms, and, therefore, the management of the patient and the focus of the dysarthria therapy may vary with subsequent exacerbations and remissions.

G. Recommended Readings

Blackwood, H. D., LaPointe, L. L., Holzapple, P., Pohlman, K., & Graham, L. F. (1991). Lexical-semantic abilities of individuals with multiple sclerosis and aphasia. In T. E. Prescott, (Ed.). *Clinical aphasiology* (Vol. 18). Austin, TX: Pro-Ed.

Darley, F. L., Aronson, A. E., & Brown, J. R. (1975). *Motor speech disorders.* Philadelphia: W.B. Saunders.

Darley, F. L., Brown, J.R., & Goldstein, N. P. (1972). Dysarthria in multiple sclerosis. *Journal of Speech & Hearing Research, 15,* 229–245.

Hier, D. B. (1991). Demyelinating diseases. In M. A. Samuels, (Ed.). *Manual of neurology: Diagnosis and therapy* (4th ed., pp. 266–274) Boston/Toronto: Little, Brown.

Panitch, H. S. (1992). Interferons in multiple sclerosis, a review of the evidence. *Drugs, 44*(6), 946–962.

Schienberg, L. C. & Holland, N. J. (Eds.). *Multiple sclerosis: A guide for patients and their families* (2nd ed.). New York: Raven Press.

Vogel, D., & Miller, L. (1991). A top-down approach to treatment of dysarthric speech. In D. Vogel & M. P. Cannito (Eds.). *Treating disordered speech motor control: For clinicians by clinicians* (Vol. 6., pp. 87–109) Austin, TX: Pro-Ed.

Three Swings. Hoping for a home run against multiple sclerosis. (1993, May) *Scientific American*, 128–129.

VI. WILSON'S DISEASE

A. Definition/Cause. Wilson's disease is an autosomal recessive familial metabolic disorder with abnormal copper metabolism that produces deposits of copper and consequent degeneration of the liver and basal ganglia. The onset of symptoms usually occurs between the ages of 10–40 years.

B. General Features, Symptoms, and Signs

1. **Younger patients** tend to have a rapidly progressive course of either Parkinsonian rigidity and bradykinesia or a hyperkinetic syndrome with athetosis.

2. **Older patients** have a less severe and slow progressive course with intention tremor, dysphagia, and dysarthria.

3. **Liver damage** may produce hepatic encephalopathy and result in confusion, inattention, and lethargy.

4. There is an appearance of Kaiser-Fleshier rings of the cornea (*see* Glossary).

5. Wilson's disease is diagnosed when decreased serum copper and ceruloplasm levels are discovered along with decreased excretion of copper in the urine.

C. Features, Symptoms, and Signs of Communication Impairment

1. S.A.K. Wilson, for whom the condition was named, reported **dysarthria** to be a cardinal feature. If the disease goes untreated, the speech deteriorates to the point of mutism.

2. Features of the dysarthric speech are reduced pitch variability or stress, lack of precision in producing consonants, irregular articulatory breakdown, prolonged intervals, equal spacing of syllables or words, slow rate; and a phonatory pattern involving low pitch, harsh voice and vocal strain, monopitch, and monoloudness. This dysarthria is a mixture of spastic, ataxic, and hypokinetic components.

D. Pharmacologic Treatment

1. **D-Penicillamine (Cupremine®),** the drug of choice, mobilizes copper from all body tissues, increases the excretion of copper, and ultimately arrests the progression of the disease.

   D-Penicillamine must be taken throughout life to control the symptoms of Wilson's disease.

   a. **Desired effect** is retardation of the progression of the disease.

   b. **Undesirable effects** are **nausea, vomiting, skin rash, impaired sense of smell, arthralgia (joint pain) leukopenia (reduction in the number of white blood cells),** and **thrombocytopenia (reduction of the number of platelets in the blood leading to spontaneous bruising and prolonged bleeding after injury). Optic neuropathy** and **nephrotic syndrome** (*see* Glossary) may be present.

2. **Triethylenetramine dihydrocloride** has been suggested for use by patients with serious toxic reactions to **D-Penicillamine.**

E. Effects of the Drugs on Communication

Although pharmacologic therapy appears to retard progression of Wilson's disease, there is a lack of evidence to suggest that it has a positive effect on communication. One exception was reported in an article by Berry et al. (1974) in which pharmacologic (D-Penicillamine) and dietary treatment produced a significant remission of dysarthric signs.

F. Alternatives to Pharmacologic Treatment

1. **Diet modification.** A diet low in copper (less than 1.5 mg/day) may decrease the requirement for **D-Penicillamine.**

2. **Speech therapy** may improve speech intelligibility.

G. Recommended Readings

Berry, W. R., Darley, F. L., Aronson, A. E., & Goldstein, N. P. (1974). Dysarthria in Wilson's disease. *Journal of Speech and Hearing Research, 17*(2), 169–183.

Darley, F. L., Aronson, A. E., & Brown, J. R. (1975). *Motor speech disorders.* Philadelphia: W.B. Saunders.

Helme, R. D. (1991). Movement disorders. In M. A. Samuels (Ed.), *Manual of neurologic therapeutics with essentials of diagnosis* (4th ed., pp. 316–334). Boston/Toronto: Little, Brown.

Wilson, S. A. K. (1912). Progressive lenticular degeneration: A familial nervous disease associated with cirrhosis of the liver. *Brain, 34,* 295–509.

VII. CEREBRAL PALSY (STATIC ENCEPHALOPATHY)

A. Definition/Cause

Cerebral palsy is a multiply handicapping motor dysfunction caused by brain abnormality resulting from maldevelopment or damage occurring before, during, or shortly after birth. A common cause is hypoxic-ischemic insult (*see* Glossary) or cerebral hemorrhage in the perinatal period.

B. General Features, Symptoms, and Signs

The group of disorders that is cerebral palsy may be classified by neurologic signs into spastic, choreoathetotic, ataxic, and mixed varieties. The motor findings associated with cerebral palsy may not be manifested until the second year of life.

1. **Spasticity** in cerebral palsy is a hyperactive stretch reflex often resulting in abnormal postures, contractures, and abnormalities of mobility, a jerkiness of movement.

2. **Athetosis** is an abnormal amount of arrhythmic, involuntary movements.

3. **Rigidity** is the increased resistance to passive motion producing slowness and decreased facility of voluntary movements.

4. **Ataxia** refers to difficulty maintaining balance with incoordination and clumsiness of movement.

5. **Sensory deficits.** Visual deficits may be evident, and there is a high incidence of conductive and sensorineural hearing loss. Frequently, either a diminished or hypersensitive response to tactile stimulation, seizures, and disordered body sensations associated with posture and movement may be noted.

6. **Physical disabilities** and **failure in attempts to perform activities of daily living** are common.

C. Features, Symptoms, and Signs of Communication Impairment

1. Poor oral and respiratory-phonatory motor control underlie the dysarthria associated with cerebral palsy. There is impairment of respiration, phonation, resonance, articulation, and prosody leading to disordered speech intelligibility.

2. Persons diagnosed with cerebral palsy often demonstrate language and cognitive deficits.

D. Pharmacologic Treatment

A variety of drugs are used for spasticity and cerebellar disorders.

1. **Baclofen (Lioresal®), dantrolene (Dantrium®), and diazepam (Valium®)** are prescribed to decrease spasticity. (*See* Amyotrophic Lateral Sclerosis, Multiple Sclerosis).

2. For patients with spasticity who do not respond to **baclofen, dantrolene,** or **diazepam,** or a combination of **phenytoin (Dilantin®),** an anticonvulsant (*see* Epilepsy), and **chlorpromazine hydrochloride (Thorazine®),** an antipsychotic agent (*see* Schizophrenia), may be beneficial.

a. **Desired effect** is decrease of spasticity.

b. **Undesirable effects** of **baclofen** are **drowsiness, hallucinations, nightmares, mania, depression, anxiety** and **confusion.** Side effects of **phenytoin** are **sedation, blurred vision,**

gastrointestinal disturbance, ataxia, vertigo, dizziness, diplopia, skin rash, and **tremor.** More severe side effects are **delayed cardiac conduction, arrythmias, hepatitis, aplastic anemia** and **arthralgia** (*see* Glossary). **Undesirable effects** of **chlorpromazine hydrochloride** are **sedation, constipation, skin rash, blurred vision,** and **weight gain.** More adverse side effects are **akinesia** (*see* Glossary), **lowered seizure threshold, tardive dyskinesia, Parkinsonism, agranulocytosis,** and **neuroleptic malignant syndrome (NMS)** (*see* Glossary).

3. Medical therapy for **cerebellar dysfunction** is disappointing. Many drugs have been used, and others are being tried with little or no reproducible benefit. **Isoniazid (INH)** has been reported by some authors to decrease symptoms of cerebellar disorder, but other authors have not confirmed the benefit of INH (*see* Multiple Sclerosis).

   a. **Desired effect.** Decrease of symptoms of cerebellar dysfunction.

   b. **Undesirable effects.** A high incidence of **hepatotoxicity** has been reported for patients taking this drug.

E. Effects of the Drugs on Communication

1. There has been no documented improvement in communication as a result of drug therapy for cerebellar dysfunction.

2. Impaired concentration and memory, and dysarthria have been reported as effects of drug treatment.

F. Alternatives to Pharmacologic Treatment

1. **Individual peripheral nerve blockade** may be necessary for relief of dystonia and abnormal postures in some patients. If this procedure is successful in eliminating or reducing symptoms, a permanent nerve block may be recommended.

2. **Physical therapy** may be prescribed to prevent contractures in spasticity and to reduce the tremor of cerebellar dysfunctioning.

3. **Electrical brain stimulation**

4. **Lesioning of the ventrolateral thalamus** may be successful in alleviating certain cerebellar tremors.

5. **Speech therapy** may improve speech production. In cases of severe dysarthria, augmentative communicative devices will be needed.

G. Recommended Readings

Helme, R. D. (1991). Movement disorders. In M. A. Samuels (Ed.), *Manual of neurology: Diagnosis and therapy* (4th ed. pp. 316–334). Boston/Toronto: Little, Brown.
McDonald, E. T. (1987). Cerebral palsy: Its nature, pathogenesis and management. In E. T. McDonald (Ed.), *Treating cerebral palsy*: For clinicians by clinicians (Vol. 4., pp. 1–19). Austin, TX: Pro-Ed.

VIII. HUNTINGTON'S DISEASE (HUNTINGTON'S CHOREA)

"The heredity chorea, as I shall call it, is confined to certain and fortunately few families, and has been transmitted to them, a heirloom from generations away back in the dim past. It is spoken of by those in whose veins the seeds are known to exist, with a kind of horror, and not at all alluded to except to the dire necessity when it is mentioned as 'that disorder.' It is attended generally by all the symptoms of common chorea, only in an aggravated degree, hardly ever manifesting itself until adult or middle life and then coming on gradually but surely increasing by degrees and often occupying years in its development, until the hapless sufferer is but a quivering wreck of his former self."

George Huntington (1872)

A. Definition/Cause

1. Huntington's Disease is an **inherited, autosomal dominant disorder** characterized by degeneration in the striatum (the caudate and putamen). The defective gene is located near the tip of chromosome 4 and is inherited by all Huntington's patients. No specific enzyme or metabolic defect has been discovered that is responsible for cell death leading to Huntington's disease.

2. **Onset** usually is between ages 25–45 years, although, occasionally, the disease has been reported in children 5 years and younger. Rarely is the initial appearance after the age of 75 years.

3. The disease lasts an average of 15 years, although survival periods as short as 5 and as long as 30 years have been recorded. Death usually occurs during the middle 50s.

4. Thirty thousand people in the United States suffer from Huntington's Disease, and another 150,000 Americans are thought to be at risk. It is a relatively rare disorder, but affects all races.

5. Each child of a parent with the disease has a 50–50 chance of having inherited it. However, occasionally, individuals develop the disease without having an affected parent. When the illness begins before the age of 21 years, the father is the affected parent nearly four times as often as the mother.

> In San Luis, a fishing village on the coast of Venezuela, it is estimated that half of the population suffers from Huntington's disease. The local residents of the village have named the condition El Mal (the bad). This dense concentration of patients allowed researchers to conduct an effective search for the affected gene.

B. General Features, Symptoms, and Signs

1. There is relative overactivity of the nigral dopaminergic system and resulting chorea. **Initial symptoms** are subtle involuntary tics and twitching that may appear as fidgeting. These involuntary movements gradually evolve into a chorea with rapid, jerky, semipurposeful movements, usually of the extremities. Initially, the patient may convert the movement into purposeful or semipurposeful motion to disguise its involuntary nature. Later, the movements become grotesque contortions with flailing arms, constricting fingers, and wild jerking of the head.

2. A **dementia** develops, with apathy, impulsive and inappropriate behavior, and personality change. Eventually, patients undergo mood swings and concentration deficits, resulting in poor functioning in the environment and memory loss. Behavioral symptoms range from abusive behavior to depression, sometimes with suicide, or psychosis.

3. The patient loses interest in self-care and, subsequently, in the ability to walk and eat. In the **final stages,** the patient becomes severely demented and bedridden.

4. Early in the disease, CT and MRI results may appear normal, but soon reveal the hallmark feature of the disease—enlargement of the frontal horns of the ventricles due to atrophy of the caudate nucleus. The putamen and, to a lesser extent, the globus pallidus are shrunken, but the brainstem and cerebellum appear normal.

C. Features, Symptoms, and Signs of Communication Impairment

1. A highly variable pattern of interference with articulation, episodes of hypernasality, harshness, breathiness, and unplanned variations in loudness occur. Speech impairment ranges from little or no dysarthria in cases where the movements are in the limbs and body only, to severely impaired, unintelligible speech. The speech may be disrupted by sudden movements of the respiratory muscles, tongue, and face. Prosody may be altered significantly as the patient attempts to avoid and compensate for the interruptions. Phonemes and intervals between words are prolonged, stress is equalized, and there are inappropriate silences. Speech is classified as hyperkinetic dysarthria.

2. Dementia is of the frontal lobe variety as described above. Apathy may produce apparent impaired memory function and diminished language use evolves into muteness in the later stages of the disease.

D. Pharmacologic Treatment

There is no definitive treatment for the neuronal degeneration. In the early stages, involuntary movements may be partially suppressed with dopamine depletion or dopamine receptor blockade.

1. **Antipsychotics (Psychotropics, Neuroleptics)** are a group of drugs that block dopamine receptors.

   a. **Haloperidol (Haldol®)** is the most commonly used neuroleptic for dopamine blockade in patients with movement disorders.
      (1) **Desired effect** is suppression of choreiform movements and control of impulsive and agitated behavior.
      (2) **Undesirable effects.** Mild side effects are **drowsiness, hypotension, blurred vision, dry mouth, and constipation.** More severe side effects are **Parkinsonism (rigidity of extremities, tremors); akathisia (restlessness with constant movement especially of the legs);** and **tardive**

dyskinesia with facial grimacing; eye-rolling; and spasm of neck muscles (*see* Psychiatric Disorders).

b. Other neuroleptics prescribed are **chlorpromazine (Thorazine®)** and **thioridazine (Mellaril®).** The side effects of these drugs are similar to those of Haloperidol. (*See* Psychiatric Disorders for desired and possible undesirable effects).

c. Reserpine (Serpasil®, Sandril®). Reserpine depletes the stores of dopamine from the nerve endings in the central nervous system.
  (1) Desired effect is decreased dopamine receptor activity, leading to reduction of symptoms.
  (2) Undesirable effects. Orthostatic hypotension is a major side effect, however, patients usually develop tolerance within a few weeks. They are warned to rise slowly to avoid lightheadedness and syncope (fainting) during that time. Reserpine also causes **depression.**

d. Tetrabenazine (Nitoman®) also depletes the stores of dopamine from nerve endings in the central nervous system. This drug is not yet available in the United States.
  (1) Desired effect is decreased dopamine receptor activity leading to reduction of symptoms.
  (2) Undesirable effects. Parkinsonism, drowsiness, and **depression** are common side effects. **Anxiety, insomnia,** and **akathisia** can occur but are less common.

E. Effects of the Drugs on Communication

1. There is no evidence of reduction of symptoms affecting communication as a result of drug therapy.

2. Tardive dyskinesia, a side effect of haloperidol, causes communication impairment (*see* Psychiatric Disorders).

F. Alternatives to Pharmacologic Treatment

1. Genetic counseling. There is no cure for Huntington's disease, and the emphasis is on prevention. Because 50% of the offspring of Huntington's patients will inherit the disease, genetic counseling is advised. Unfortunately, the mean age of onset is 35 years, and persons may not be aware of their predisposition to Huntington's disease before making the decision to become parents.

The knowledge that the locus for Huntington's disease was on chromosome 4 quickly led to a test to determine whether offspring of carriers—either in utero or already born—had inherited the gene itself, and would develop Huntington's disease. However, the test requires analysis of blood samples from several members of the same family with and without the defective gene, and this often is difficult to achieve. Family members with the condition may deny it initially and later, when dementia develops, may not be cooperative. Those who are not yet clinically affected may be concerned about their own risk and may not want to know their ultimate fate. Therefore, they also may be unwilling to cooperate. Disruption of family life, depression, and even suicide could result from the knowledge of future disease. Furthermore, the false positives that may occur with this analysis may make it an unreliable predictor of the disease.

It took six teams of workers from ten institutions an additional 10 years to identify the gene on chromosome 4 that is actually responsible for Huntington's disease. Each time the gene is transmitted, the number of replications of the gene may expand. This phenomenon has been demonstrated in a number of genetically transmitted diseases. It appears that the greater the expansion, the earlier the onset; but how the gene actually causes Huntington's disease is still not known, and treatment or cure is not likely in the near future.

2. **Speech, voice, and language therapy.** The efficacy of therapy for the dysarthria and dementia of Huntington's disease is uncertain. Management involves advising patients and their caregivers of how to obtain the most effective communication possible.

G. Recommended Readings

Horgan, J. (1993, June). Eugenics revisited. The Huntington's disease saga: A cautionary tale. *Scientific American,* 126.
Jerome, R. (1993, May/June). Huntington's cornered. *The Sciences,* 7.

IX. GILLES DE LA TOURETTE'S SYNDROME (TOURETTE'S SYNDROME; TOURETTE'S DISORDER)

A. Definition/Cause

1. **Tics** are quick, coordinated, repetitive movements. Unlike tremors, they are not rhythmic and unlike the chorea of Huntington's disease, they are not irregular, nonrepetitive, or quasi-purposeful movements.

2. Tourette's syndrome is characterized by **multiple motor** and **one or more vocal tics** that can appear either simultaneously or at different periods during the illness. The disorder is common among first degree biologic relatives.

3. Tourette's syndrome may begin as early as one year of age. The median age at onset is 7 years. For the greatest majority of patients, onset occurs by age 14 years.

B. General Features, Symptoms, and Signs

1. The tics that characterize Tourette's syndrome begin in childhood and worsen intermittently and variably during the life of the individual.

2. Tics may occur several times a day, almost every day, or intermittently throughout a period of more than one year. They involve the head, neck, and shoulders, predominantly, but may also involve the torso and upper and lower limbs.

3. Tongue protrusions, squatting, sniffing, excessive hopping or skipping, and twirling when walking are observable signs of Tourette's syndrome. Retracing steps and other obsessive-compulsive behaviors may occur.

4. In nearly 50% of cases, the first symptoms to appear are bouts of a single tic. Eye blinking is the most frequent early symptom.

5. Tourette's syndrome can cause the inability to coordinate a swallow.

6. Although, usually, Tourette's syndrome is a lifelong condition, periods of remission lasting from weeks to years have been reported. In some cases, the severity and frequency of symptoms diminish during adolescence and adulthood, and in other cases, the symptoms last until or throughout adulthood.

C. Features, Symptoms, and Signs of Communication Impairment

1. Vocal tics include various involuntary sounds such as clicks, grunts, yelps, barks, sniffs, coughs, screams, snorts, and stutterings that interrupt the flow of speech. Echolalia has been observed. Coprolalia, the uttering of obscenities, is present in up to 50% of cases.

2. Reduced voice volume and velar and lingual dystonia affecting voice and speech have been noted.

D. Pharmacologic Treatment

Dopamine blockers such as haloperidol and pimozide have been prescribed.

1. Haloperidol (Haldol®)

a. Desired effects are control of tics and coprolalia.

b. Undesirable effects: Skin rash, dizziness, weakness, agitation, insomnia, loss of appetite, indigestion, gastrointestinal disorders, and **urinary retention** are mild side effects. More serious side effects are **tremors, akathisia (restlessness), facial grimacing, eye rolling,** and **spasm of neck muscles.** Chronic use of **Haldol** can result in **eye damage (deposits in cornea, lens, or retina)** and **tardive dyskinesia** (*see* Psychiatric Disorders).

2. Pimozide (Orap®) is related to major tranquilizers used to relieve hallucinations and delusions occurring in schizophrenia (*see* Psychiatric Disorders). Tourette's syndrome is approved by the FDA (*see* Glossary) as the indication for Pimozide.

a. Desired effects are relief from tics and other symptoms of Tourette's syndrome.

b. **Undesirable effects** include **skin rash, tremors,** and other **Parkinsonian symptoms, tardive dyskinesia, sedation, headache,** and **hypotension.** Additional side effects are **constipation, decreased libido, amenorrhea** (*see* Glossary), **weight gain,** and **anticholinergic effects (dry mouth, urinary retention, blurred vision).**

3. **Clonidine (Catapres®)**

   a. **Desired effect** is control of abnormal movements.

   b. **Undesirable effects. Drowsiness, dry nose and mouth, constipation, decreased heart rate, and mild orthostatic hypotension** are common. Additional side effects are **skin rash, headache, dizziness, fatigue, anxiety, nervousness, dryness and burning of the eyes, painful parotid gland, nausea, vomiting, weight gain,** and **urinary retention.**

   Overdose of clonidine can cause **drowsiness, weakness, slow pulse, vomiting, low blood pressure,** and **stupor progressing to coma.** **Marked drowsiness** and **exaggerated reduction of blood pressure** can occur when alcohol is taken concurrently with clonidine. Possible effects of long term use are **tolerance, weight gain due to salt and fluid retention,** and **temporary sexual impotence.**

E. Effects of the Drugs on Communication

1. Successful drug therapy controls the vocal tics and the coprolalia that interfere with communication.

2. The medication can produce side effects that have an impact upon communication.

F. Alternatives To Pharmacologic Treatment

No alternative treatment has proven to be wholly effective for eliminating or controlling the symptoms of Tourette's syndrome. Originally, it was thought that the bizarre behavior was psychiatric in origin. **Psychotherapy** has yielded only a limited degree of temporary success.

G. Recommended Reading:

Licamele, W., & Goldberg, R. L. (1988). Tourette syndrome. *American Family Physician, 37*(4), 115–119.

CHAPTER

3

Language Specific
Neurologic Disorders

This chapter covers neurologic disorders that may affect language. For each disorder, we provide a definition and cause; discuss the general features, symptoms, and signs; describe the features, symptoms, and signs of language impairment associated with each disorder; list pharmacologic treatment for each disorder; and discuss the influence drug treatment may have on language.

I. STROKE

A. Definition/Cause(s)

1. Stroke is a sudden or rapid onset of a focal neurologic deficit caused by cerebrovascular disease. Blood supply to the brain is disrupted, resulting in disturbance of function to the part of the brain that is nourished by the damaged blood vessel.

2. Approximately 500,000 new strokes occur each year and about 150,000 people die as a result. It is the third leading cause of death in the United States and is the leading cause of disability.

3. Eighty-five percent of strokes are due to **cerebral ischemia**. The degree of infarction following occlusion of an artery to the brain depends on the degree of reduction of blood flow, the duration of ischemia, and the adequacy of the collateral blood flow.

    a. One cause of ischemic stroke is **cerebral thrombosis**. This is a condition in which damage to the wall of an artery from athero-sclerosis causes the blood in an artery to form a clot (thrombus) within the lumen of the artery. The thrombus obstructs the blood flow to the tissue it supplies, producing an ischemic stroke.

    b. **Cerebral embolism** is a second cause of ischemic stroke. It is a condition in which some particular material, usually a blood clot, but sometimes fat, air, amniotic fluid, or a foreign body, is carried by the blood from one point in the circulation to lodge in another, thus, blocking the flow of blood through the artery. The most common source of embolism is the heart.

4. **Hemorrhagic Strokes.** Intracerebral hemorrhage most commonly is caused by hypertension-induced vascular disease. Subarachnoid hemorrhage usually occurs as a result of a ruptured congenital aneurysm or arteriovenous malformation.

B. General Features, Symptoms, and Signs

1. A stroke produces **sudden loss of neurologic function** including motor control, sensory perception, vision, language, visuospatial function, and memory. There may be fluctuating severity of the neurologic deficits for the first few hours. This is referred to as a **stuttering onset.** Some patients experience stroke symptoms that last for minutes or hours, and then symptoms resolve. This is referred to as a **transient ischemic attack** (TIA) (*see* Glossary). TIAs indicate a high risk of subsequent stroke.

2. **Signs of cerebral hemorrhage** are sudden onset of headache that grows worse rapidly and is associated with steady progression of neurologic signs. Increased cranial pressure as the hemorrhage enlarges may produce vomiting.

C. Features, Symptoms, and Signs of Communication Impairment

Strokes can cause a wide variety of communication impairment: for example, aphasia, dysarthria, and dementia. The type and severity of the impaired communication are dependent upon the brain structures involved.

D. Pharmacologic Treatment for Stroke Prevention

1. **Anticoagulants** are prescribed for patients who are at continued risk for clotting. **Heparin** is an intravenous anticoagulant administered at the very onset of stroke. **Warfarin (Coumadin®)** may be used for long-term, oral therapy. It interferes with the chemicals circulating in the blood that contribute to clotting of the blood.

   a. **Desired effects.** These drugs are used to inhibit blood coagulation and, therefore, prevent thromboembolic strokes. They are used most commonly when the risk of embolic stroke is high: for example, in cases in which cardiac disease predisposes the presence of blood clots inside the heart.

   b. **Undesirable effects** are **hemorrhage; thrombocytopenia (reduction of the number of platelets in the blood resulting in prolonged bleeding), hematoma, necrosis**, and **gastrointestinal disturbance.** Annually, 1–2% of patients on warfarin experience a **hemorrhage** severe enough to require transfusion or a **intracranial hematoma** that can be fatal. The high risk of severe complications must be balanced carefully with the benefit of using the drug.

2. **Platelet antiaggregant agents.** Platelets, the agents in the blood that contribute to the formation of clots, may adhere to damaged blood vessel walls and begin the chain reaction that produces a thrombus. Antiplatelet medications diminish platelet aggregation and, therefore, prevent the clots that can lead to stroke. Generally, these drugs are not as effective as anticoagulants for inhibiting blood clotting, but the risk is lower for hemorrhage than it is with anticoagulant drugs.

   a. **Aspirin (ASA).** Although available over-the-counter (OTC), and not a prescription drug, aspirin is discussed here because it is used frequently for stroke prevention. Aspirin has been shown to decrease the incidence of stroke in patients who are at high risk because of previous stroke, TIA, or other manifestations of atherosclerosis, for example, heart attack. The morbidity rate for aspirin therapy is relatively low. Although some physicians recommend aspirin for all persons in an age group at high risk for atherosclerosis, prevention of heart attack and ischemic stroke must be weighed against the possibility of hemorrhagic stroke. Enteric coated aspirin often is recommended to prevent gastrointestinal distress.

(1) **Desired effect** is prevention of initial or subsequent stroke

(2) **Undesirable effects. Skin rash, nasal discharge, stomach irritation, gastrointestinal ulceration and subsequent hemorrhage, asthma; unusual bruising due to impaired platelet function, hepatitis with jaundice; and activation of peptic ulcer, with or without hemorrhage** are side effects of aspirin. In addition, **kidney damage** can occur if aspirin is used in large doses or for a prolonged period of time.

Overdose of aspirin can result in **gastrointestinal disturbance, tinnitis and impaired hearing, dizziness, sweating, stupor, fever, deep and rapid breathing, muscle twitching, delirium, hallucinations**, and **convulsions.**

b. **Ticlopidine (Ticlid®)** is indicated to prevent recurrence of stroke in patients who are at increased risk for stroke and who have failed to respond or are allergic to aspirin. Patients who continue to experience TIAs while taking aspirin, and who, in the judgment of their treating physician, are at considerable risk for stroke may be offered ticlopidine to reduce the risk.

(1) **Desired effects** are prevention of TIAs and stroke.

(2) **Undesirable effects** are **moderate dyspepsia** and **diarrhea** that may be averted if ticlopidine is taken with meals or discontinued gradually. Side effects usually occur early in the treatment. The most significant problem is bone marrow depression producing decreased white blood cells necessary to fight infection **(neutropenia** or **agranulocytosis),** with decreased platelets (agranulocytosis) occurring within the first 3 months of therapy. For this reason, a biweekly monitoring of the complete blood count (CBC) is recommended during that time.

(3) **Ticlopidine** should not be used in combination with certain drugs, for example, **cimetidine (Tagamet®), aspirin, warfarin, or nonsteroidal anti-inflammatory agents** unless there are specific or compelling reasons to do so, for example, occasional pain.

3. **Thrombolytic Agents** are used to degrade clots that have already formed. The most commonly used thrombolytic drugs are **streptokinase, urokinase,** and **anistreplase (Eminase®).**

> The venoms of pit vipers, for example, rattlesnakes, copperheads and cottonmouth water moccasins, are thrombolytic agents. Venoms from selected species of pit vipers are being investigated for treatment of acute stroke.

a. **Desired effect** is the degrading of blood clots in the setting of acute stroke.

b. **Undesirable effects** are bleeding and bruising. Bleeding into the brain may occur; thus there is a delicate balance between administering too little and too much of a thrombolytic agent.

Recently, in an investigation of an experimental drug that mimics the illicit PCP, it was found that **Selfotel**® appears to halt the disastrous chemical chain reaction that destroys cells after stroke interferes with the blood supply. It seems to stop the self-destructive response after the clot disrupts the supply of oxygen to the brain. The most troublesome side effect of **Selfotel**® reported to date involves **hallucinations** that are similar to those triggered by PCP.

---

3. Reactive depression is a common consequence of stroke. For a discussion of antidepressant therapy *see* Psychiatric Disorders.

E. Effects of the Drugs on Communication

The drugs used for stroke prevention have no direct effect on communication. Indirectly, these medications affect communication by preventing the stroke that underlies the communication disorder.

1. Pharmacologic Treatment for Aphasia

a. In the past few years, some investigators have hypothesized that the dopamine agonist, **bromocriptine**, has a beneficial effect on recovery from aphasia, particularly, transcortical motor aphasia. The rationale underlying this hypothesis is that impaired initiation of speech production is similar to the impaired initiation of motor activity in Parkinson's disease. This indicates that enhanced dopaminergic activity might be helpful in alleviating symptoms. To date, results of most studies conducted to determine the effects of bromocriptine on recovery from aphasia have demonstrated no positive effect. Recently, results of a double-blind placebo controlled study of 15 nonfluent aphasic patients, indicated no difference in the performance of a sizable number of language tasks between patients taking bromocriptine and those taking placebos. *See* Parkinson's disease, for desired and undesirable effects of bromocriptine.

b. **Amphetamine** has been used in an attempt to facilitate recovery from aphasia following stroke. Investigators have reported

varying levels of success with some patients. *See* Attention
Deficit Hyperactivity Disorder, for desired and undesirable
affects of amphetamine.

F. Alternative Treatments

1. **Speech and Language Therapy**. Several investigations have
demonstrated that speech therapy is an efficacious treatment for
patients with aphasia. In addition, speech therapy for motor speech
disorders following stroke has been reported to be beneficial.
Counseling caregivers of patients with dementia subsequent to stroke
and providing suggestions on how to achieve the most effective communication possible has been beneficial as well.

2. **Other rehabilitative services**, for example, physical and occupa-
tional therapy, are efficacious for stroke rehabilitation.

G. Recommended Readings

Albert, M.L., Bachman, D. L., Morgan, A., & Helm-Estabrooks, N. (1989)
Pharmacotherapy for aphasia. *Neurology, 38*, 877–879.

Bachman, D. L., & Morgan, A. (1988). The role of pharmacotherapy in the
treatment of aphasia: Preliminary results. *Aphasiology, 2*, 225–228.

Gupta, S., Mlcoch. A., Scolaro, C., & Moritz, T. (1994). Bromocriptine treatment of non-fluent aphasia. *Veterans Administration Merit Review
Investigation.*

MacLennan, D. L., Nicholas, L. E., Morley, G. K., & Brookshire, R. H. (1991).
The effects of bromocriptine in a man with transcortical motor aphasia. In
T. E. Prescott (Ed.), *Clinical aphasiology* (Vol. 20, pp. 145–156). Austin,
TX: Pro-Ed.

Salvatore, A., Vogel, D. Carter, J. E., & Leitgen-Pfannstiel, J. (1993,
November). *Independent evaluation of the effects of bromocriptine on
aphasia.* Paper presented at American Speech-Language-Hearing
Association Convention, Anaheim.

Vogel, D., Carter, J. E., & Faber, R. (November, 1992). Neuropharmacology for
the speech-language pathologist: An update. Short Course presented at
American Speech-Language-Hearing Association Convention, San
Antonio, TX.

Walker-Batson, D., Devous, M. D., Curtis, S. S., Unwin, D. H., & Greenlee, R.
(1991). Response to amphetamine to facilitate recovery from aphasia subsequent to stroke. In T. E. Prescott (Ed.), *Clinical aphasiology* (Vol. 20, pp.
137–143). Austin, TX: Pro-Ed.

Walker-Batson, D., Unwin, H. , Curtis, S., Allen, E., Wood, M., Smith, P.,
Devous, M. D., Reynolds, S., & Greenlee, R. G. (1991). Use of amphetamine in the treatment of aphasia. *Restorative Neurology and Neuroscience,
4*, 4–50.

Wertz, R. T., Weiss, D, G., Aten, J. L., Brookshire, R. H., Garcia-Bunuel, L. M., Holland, A. L., Kurtzke, J. F., LaPointe, L. L., Milianti, F. J., Brannegan, R., Greenbaum, H., Marshall, R.C., Vogel, D., Carter, J. E., Barnes, N. S., & Goodman, R. (1986). Comparison of clinic, home and deferred language treatment for aphasia. A Veterans Administration Cooperative Study. *Archives of Neurology, 43*, 653–658.

II. EPILEPSY (SEIZURE DISORDER)

A. Definition/Cause

Epilepsy is a chronic disorder characterized by recurring seizures that last from a few seconds to several minutes and require specific drugs for their prevention and control.

1. The actual seizure is due to a **sudden, abnormal, excessive, electrical discharge** within the brain. In primary epilepsy, the basic cause is unknown, and no focus of abnormal electrical activity can be identified in the brain. There may be a genetic predisposition.

2. **In secondary epilepsy** a focus of abnormal electrical activity can be identified somewhere in the cerebral cortex or the hippocampus/amygdala complex in the temporal lobe. This abnormal focus fires spontaneously, and occasionally "recruits" surrounding normal neurons to discharge synchronously, producing a seizure. The seizure can be a complication of developmental abnormalities, head injury, bacterial meningitis or encephalitis, or it may be associated with stroke, cerebral palsy, brain tumor, or hydrocephalus.

B. General Features, Symptoms and Signs

1. Principal types of epilepsy include **tonic-clonic, absence,** and **complex partial seizures.**

   a. **Tonic-clonic** seizures are sudden attacks that begin with an involuntary cry, followed by loss of consciousness and falling; violent convulsive movements of the head, trunk, and extremities; excessive salivation; and loss of bladder and/or bowel control. The individual awakens a few minutes after the seizure and is dazed and confused for a period of minutes or hours.

   b. **Absence** seizures typically begin between 2–12 years of age. There is a sudden lapse of consciousness that lasts no more than 30 seconds. The individual exhibits a blank stare and appears oblivious of the surroundings. There is no convulsion and no fall although there may be a minor twitching of an eyelid or facial muscle, chewing movements, or a jerk of a hand or arm. Episodes may occur infrequently or as often as more than 100 times per day. Following each episode, the individual resumes normal functioning and does not remember the seizure.

c. **Complex partial** seizures (psychomotor; temporal lobe epilepsy) comprise 40% of all epilepsies. Some begin with an "aura" associated with distorted vision, unpleasant odors or tastes, visual and auditory hallucinations, and bizarre illusions. The individual may walk aimlessly, talk irrationally, and engage in purposeless behaviors such as striking the wall. The behavior may appear purposeful, but may be carried out ineffectively. For example, the patient may arise from a chair, walk across the room to pull the curtains open, then became tangled up in the curtains. After the seizure, the individual is confused and has no recollection of the event.

C. Features, Symptoms, and Signs of Communication Impairment

1. **Complex partial** seizures precipitate alterations of behavior that involve speech, memory, hearing, and emotional responses. Aphasia, which usually is transient, may follow a seizure.

2. **Landau-Kleffner Syndrome (Childhood Aphasia)** is a condition in which, following seizure, there is an acute onset of language dysfunction in children whose language, previously, was normal. Usually, age of onset is between 3 and 9 years. An auditory comprehension deficit described as a verbal auditory agnosia is a feature of Landau-Kleffner syndrome. The natural course of this childhood aphasia ranges from nearly complete language recovery in a minority of patients, to intermediate or severe dysfunction in the majority.

D. Pharmacologic Treatment

1. The **primary goal of drug therapy** for seizures is complete prevention. The most appropriate anticonvulsant drug is selected based on the patient's seizure type, age, and gender. The dose of the drug is progressively increased until the seizures are controlled and the patient is free of unacceptable side effects. Usually, if a first drug is ineffective, it is discontinued and another drug is tried. Ideally, patients should be treated with a single anticonvulsant, or, at the most, two. All anticonvulsive drugs have toxic effects when taken in large doses.

a. **Phenytoin (Dilantin®)** suppresses repetitive firing of normal neurons with connections to the neurons involved in the seizure, and is used to control all except absence seizures.

   (1) **Desired effects.** Control of tonic-clonic and complex-partial seizures.

   (2) **Undesirable effects** are many and include a **measles-like rash** within the first 2 weeks of administration, **high fever, headache, dizziness, insomnia,** and **fatigue. Additional, milder effects** are **overgrowth of gum tissues** (most common in children) and **excessive growth of body hair** (most common in young girls). Serious side effects of phenytoin are **drug induced hepatitis, drug-induced nephritis with acute kidney failure, severe skin reactions,** and **generalized enlargement of lymph glands. Bone marrow depression** (*see* Glossary), **confusion, ataxia, joint pain and swelling,** and **elevated blood sugar due to inhibition of insulin release** are additional uncommon side effects.

b. **Phenobarbital (Luminal®)** is a barbiturate used as an anticonvulsant to control all types of tonic-clonic and partial seizures as well as febrile seizures (seizures that accompany fevers) in childhood. How **phenobarbital** works is not completely understood. Conceivably, it could block the transmission of nerve impulses, producing a sedative effect and suppressing the spread of neuroimpulses responsible for seizures. Barbiturates were early anticonvulsants, but now are used less frequently because of their persistent sedative effect. This effect is not present in most anticonvulsants.

   (1) **Desired effects**. Control of tonic-clonic and partial-complex seizures.

   (2) **Undesirable effects. Sedation**. Mild side effects are **allergic reactions**, for example, **skin rash, hives, and localized swelling of the face**. Additional side effects are **dizziness, unsteadiness, impaired vision or diplopia,** and **gastrointestinal disturbance**. More severe side effects include **drug-induced hepatitis; depression; abnormal voluntary movements,** and **deficiencies of blood cell types causing fatigue, weakness, fever, sore throat, abnormal bleeding, and bruising. Hypothermia** may occur in elderly persons.

   (3) **Phenobarbital** usually is not administered to hyperkinetic children who may experience an increase in their hyperactivity if this drug is taken. All barbiturates are avoided in the elderly, if possible, but, if they are used, small doses are

initiated and the dosage increased gradually until the patient's tolerance is determined.

c. **Carbamazepine (Tegretol®)**. The actions of carbamazepine are similar to those of **phenytoin**.
  (1) **Desired effects**. Control of tonic-clonic and complex partial seizures.
  (2) **Undesirable effects. Bone marrow depression** or **elevated liver enzymes** may occur early in the use of the drug. **Skin rash, headache, dizziness or vertigo, drowsiness, ataxia, fatigue, blurred vision, confusion, tinnitis, loss of appetite, gastrointestinal disturbance, edema, changes in skin pigmentation, hair loss, aching of muscles,** and **joint and leg cramps** are all milder side effects of carbamazepine. Serious adverse effects include severe **dermatitis, with irritation of mouth and tongue; swelling of lymph glands; kidney damage; depression; agitation; diplopia; visual hallucinations; peripheral neuritis;** and **thrombophlebitis. Latent psychosis** and **systemic lupus erythematosus** may be activated by this drug.

d. **Clonazepam (Klonipin®)**.
  (1) **Desired effects. Clonazepam** may be useful in the treatment of absence seizures.
  (2) **Undesirable effects. Sedation, ataxia, gastrointestinal disturbance,** and **hypersalivation** are side effects of clonazepam. Many of the side effects of **benzodiazepines** are also side effects of clonazepam (*see* Psychiatric Disorders).

e. **Valproic Acid (Depakote®)** may be used as the single drug in the management of patients who have both typical absence and general tonic-clonic seizures. Valproic acid was developed after the development of phenytoin and carbamazepine, and is not used as often in the initial treatment of tonic-clonic and partial complex seizures.
  (1) **Desired effect** is prevention of seizures.
  (2) **Undesirable effects. Valproic acid** produces **central nervous system depression, elevations of liver enzymes and hepatitis, gastrointestinal disturbance, drowsiness, ataxia, headache** and **skin rash. Substantial weight gain** is a common side effect.

f. **Several new anticonvulsant drugs** have been released recently or will be available soon. Table 3–1 is a list of these drugs, and their desired and undesirable effects.

TABLE 3–1. New anti-seizure (anticonvulsant) drugs.

Drug	Desired Effect(s)	Undesirable Effects	Comments
Felbamate (Felbatol®)	Control of partial and secondary generalized seizures	Insomnia, anorexia and weight loss may be persistent. Headache is common, especially in patients taking Tegretol®, but may resolve. Nausea, dizziness, ataxia may resolve. Not linked to neutropenia, agranulocytosis, hepatotoxicity. Aplastic anemia.	Must be taken in several doses per day. Because it has been discovered that felbamate may cause aplastic anemia, it has been suggested that patient use be suspended unless the drug is the only agent that controls the seizures.
Gabapentin (Neurontin®)	Control of partial and secondary generalized seizures. Has no effect on the levels of other anticonvulsants.	Lethargy, drowsiness, ataxia; dizziness (uncommon).	Must be divided into four doses daily.
Lamotrigine (Lamictal®) (To be released soon)	Control of partial and secondary generalized seizures. May be useful in primary generalized seizures.	Dizziness, ataxia, drowsiness; drug interactions with other anticonvulsants.	Inhibits release of glutamate and aspartate.
Vigabatrin® (To be released soon)	Control of partial and secondary generalized seizures. May be useful in primary generalized epilepsies of childhood.	Drowsiness, dizziness. Depression in 5–15% of patients.	Increased GABA activity. Few interactions with other anticonvulsants. Must be given twice daily to decrease side effects.

History of Anticonvulsants

When sedating patients with barbiturates, it was discovered that these drugs had anticonvulsant effects. A subsequent search for anticonvulsants without these sedating effects led to the development in 1938, of **Dilantin**®. This drug remained the primary anticonvulsant for partial and generalized seizures in adults until the release of **Tegretol**® in 1974, and **Depakote**® in 1978. Then, 15 years passed until the release of **felbamate** in 1992. Unfortunately, recently it was announced that felbamate causes aplastic anemia in some patients. Therefore, it has been suggested that **all patient use be suspended** except in cases where felbamate proves to be the only drug that controls the seizures.

E. Effects of the Drugs on Communication

1. Some anticonvulsants **(phenytoin, carbamazepine)** can cause dysarthria and confusion. **Tinnitis** is a side effect of carbamazepine.

2. Improvements in language development and articulation have been reported in children diagnosed with Landau-Kleffner syndrome following treatment with anticonvulsant drugs.

F. Alternative Treatments

1. Seizures rarely require emergency intervention unless the seizure activity has resulted in life-threatening severe **hypoxia** (depletion of oxygen) or **acidosis** (abnormally high acidity of body fluids and tissues). To prevent aspiration, if vomiting occurs the patient is placed in a semiprone position with the head lowered until full consciousness is regained. Care is taken to provide an adequate airway. **Endotracheal intubation** and/or **oxygen administered by face mask** may be needed for prolonged or repetitive seizures.

2. **Speech-Language Therapy.** The aphasia following seizures in adults may be transitory and may not require treatment. However, it is likely that a child in the process of acquiring language at the time seizures occur and who demonstrates a language deficit, for example, Landau-Kleffner syndrome, will benefit from speech-language therapy.

G. Recommended Readings

Landau, W. M., & Kleffner, F. R. (1957). Syndrome of acquired aphasia with convulsive disorder in children. *Neurology, 7*, 523–530.

Long, J. W. (1993). *The essential guide to prescription drugs*. New York: Harper-Collins.

Mackey, R. W. (1992). The effects of drugs on language and learning disorders in a pediatric population. In D. Vogel (Ed.), Drug Treatment Issues: Special Division 2. *Neurophysiology and Neurogenic Speech and Language Newsletter, 2*(2). (Available from American Speech-Language Hearing Association, Rockville, MD.)

III. NEOPLASM

A. Definition/Cause

1. Approximately 8,500 deaths occur in the United States each year from primary brain tumors. Many additional deaths are due to cerebral metastases from malignant tumors elsewhere in the body.

2. The **age of peak incidence** is 45–55 years and the male/female ratio is 3:2.

3. The site of **brain neoplasm** is related to type of tumor. Primary brain tumors in children occur most often in the posterior fossa in the cerebellum. In adults, primary brain tumors occur most frequently in the cerebral hemispheres.

4. The **most common primary brain tumor** in adults is derived from connective tissue cells of the brain, the astrocytes. Astrocytomas are graded on the basis of severity of pathology from 1 thorough 4, with 4 as the most malignant. Malignant astrocytomas also may be referred to as **glioblastoma multiforme astrocytoma**. Glioblastoma multiforme grows rapidly and the prognosis is poor, with a median survival time after diagnosis of 9–12 months. Only 10–15% of patients survive more than 2 years after diagnosis.

5. **Low grade (1&2) astrocytomas** are less common than glioblastoma multiforme, perhaps, because they cause fewer symptoms. These tumors are slow growing and may remain relatively benign. It is possible, however, that they can develop into higher grade tumors.

6. **Meningiomas** are the second most common primary intracranial tumors in adults. They can arise outside the brain, itself, wherever

arachnoid cells are present. Meningiomas are benign, but they occupy space within a closed area. Therefore, they produce elevated intracranial pressure within the cranial cavity and also compress important structures including the brain, cranial nerves, and blood vessels.

7. **Cerebellar astrocytoma and medullablastoma** are the most common brain tumors in children. Usually these arise in the posterior fossa. These tumors tend to have a good response to surgical removal and radiation therapy. They are slow growing. Prognosis may be excellent.

B. General Features, Symptoms, and Signs

1. The character and rate of progression of neurologic symptoms and signs depend on the location and rate of growth of the tumor and its surrounding edema.

2. **Increased intracranial pressure** producing **headache,** sometimes with **nausea**, is common with large tumors or tumors that block the ventricular system and produce hydrocephalus.

3. **Focal seizures** and **generalized convulsions** occur in about one third of patients with cerebral tumors. These symptoms are more likely to accompany slower-growing rather than fast-growing, highly malignant tumors.

4. **Signs of cerebellar astrocytoma in infants** are irritability, vomiting, and an enlarging head (due to obstructive hydrocephalus). In older children, there may be headache with or without vomiting, incoordination, and ataxia.

C. Features, Symptoms, and Signs of Communication Impairment

The presence and type of communication impairment will depend upon the location of the tumor and the extent and involvement of the surrounding brain tissue. Aphasia or dysarthria may be observed.

D. Pharmacologic Treatment

1. **Corticosteroids**. Intracranial pressure (ICP) is increased markedly with large tumors or tumors producing cerebral edema. Steroid therapy results in a decrease of focal neurological signs, for example, **paresis** and **sensory loss, and in a reduction of headache** and **nausea**. For most patients, improvement begins within 24–48 hours after corticosteroid therapy is initiated. The maximum degree

of improvement is obtained by the fourth or fifth day and may continue for several weeks.

    a. Dexamethasone and **prednisone** are the most widely used preparations for treating cerebral edema. Dexamethasone is preferred by some patients due to its low salt-retaining side effects.

        (1) Desired effects. Decrease of focal neurological signs and reduction of headache and nausea.

        (2) Undesirable effects. *See* Table 2–3 for side effects of corticosteroids. Typically, these side effects are not considered a contraindication for prescribing the drug. In the case of a benign tumor that does not metastasize and destroy surrounding or distant tissue, and is not cancerous, treatment will be temporary and will be limited to a period prior to and for a brief time after surgery. In the case of a malignant tumor, the benefits of steroid therapy will outweigh the side effects of the drugs.

2. Osmotic Agents. Patients with brain tumor may experience a sudden dramatic increase in ICP due, for example, to hemorrhage within the tumor, with signs of cerebral herniation and imminent death. Situations that require rapid reduction of intracranial pressure are indications for therapy with osmotic agents.

    a. Mannitol (Osmitrol®), infused intravenously, can reduce brain fluid quickly and reduce ICP to about 30–60% for 2–4 hours. Unfortunately, the effects of mannitol may reverse completely within 8–12 hours after administration. Therefore, at the same time mannitol is administered, steroid therapy is started because of its sustained effects. Osmolar therapy is useful for the short term only, until surgery or steroids can be instituted.

        (1) Desired effect is reduction of intracranial pressure.

        (2) Undesirable effects. A rebound increase in ICP may occur. Additional possible adverse reactions are **headache, confusion, blurred vision, nausea**, and **cellular dehydration with resulting thirst.**

E. Effects of the Drugs on Communication

Drugs reduce intracranial pressure and, therefore, improve cognition and communication.

F. Alternatives to Pharmacologic Treatment

1. Surgery. Craniotomy is the primary therapy for most tumors in the cerebral hemispheres and the surrounding areas. During this procedure, a portion of the skull overlying the tumor is removed, the tumor is resected, and a bone flap is replaced for protective and cosmetic reasons. For deep, inaccessible lesions, needle biopsy with CT monitored stereotaxic techniques may be employed.

2. **Radiation Therapy**. In cases of glioblastoma multiforme, metastases, medullablastoma, and other responsive neoplasms, radiotherapy is delivered to the whole brain. Radiation therapy tends to prolong survival, somewhat, after surgery for glioblastoma multiforme and metastatic tumors, but eventually the tumor will prove to be fatal.

3. **Chemotherapy**. A variety of chemotherapeutic agents have been employed with some prolongation of survival.

4. **Speech-Language therapy** is palliative. The speech-language clinician attempts to identify the optimum conditions and methods for communication and counsels the patient and the patient's significant others regarding optimum communication.

G. Recommended Reading

Weiss, H. D. (1991). Neoplasms. In M.A. Samuels, (Ed.), *Manual of neurology: Diagnosis and therapy* (4th ed., pp. 216–242) Boston/Toronto: Little, Brown.

CHAPTER

4

DISORDERS OF COGNITION

This chapter covers neurologic disorders that may affect cognitive abilities. For each disorder, we provide a definition and cause; discuss the general features, symptoms and signs; describe the features, symptoms and signs of cognitive impairment associated with each disorder; list pharmacologic treatment for each disorder; and discuss the influence drug treatment may have on cognition.

I. ACQUIRED IMMUNE DEFICIENCY SYNDROME (AIDS)

A. Definition/Cause

1. The **primary cause** of Acquired Immune Deficiency Disease (AIDS) is the severe and protracted suppression of the immune system resulting from infection with the human immunodeficiency virus (HIV).

2. The term "AIDS" refers to the later stages of the HIV infection when failure of the immune system results in the development of serious and life-threatening infections and/or malignancies. The

period of time from the onset of the HIV infection to the terminal stages of AIDS varies from several months to as long as 15 years.

3. HIV has been found in human secretions and in certain body tissues.

B. General Features, Symptoms, and Signs

1. **HIV Infection.** Patients infected with HIV often develop an acute flu-like illness that includes fever, enlargement of the lymph gland, rash, and malaise. All patients recover from this but remain infected with the virus. Approximately, 5–10% of HIV infected patients progress to clinical disease each year.

   a. Neurologic disease may be the first manifestation of HIV infection.

2. **AIDS-Related Complex** (ARC). In this period, the patient develops symptoms of fever, night sweats, swollen lymph glands, persistent diarrhea and weight loss, and oral yeast infections and leukoplakia (white plaque-like thickening of the oral mucosa). There may be persistent Herpes zoster or Herpes simplex infections. Personality changes and intellectual impairment develop as part of AIDS related dementia.

3. **AIDS.** AIDS refers to the later stages of HIV infection when the failure of the immune system results in serious and life-threatening infections and malignancies. The usual interval from positive blood test to onset of AIDS is 8–11 years.

As chronic HIV infection progresses, it becomes impossible for the immune system to prevent opportunistic infections or malignancies from occurring. Consequently, a number of diseases and conditions develop. These diseases and conditions are listed in Table 4–1.

C. Features, Symptoms, and Signs of Communication Impairment

The topography of brain impairment varies considerably in AIDS patients. Some develop diffuse disorders, while others demonstrate focal impairment. Therefore, the communication impairment secondary to the underlying neurological condition experienced by patients with AIDS varies.

TABLE 4–1. Some complications associated with HIV/AIDS.

Pneumocystis Carinii Pneumonia (PCP)

Toxoplasmosis

Cryptococcosis
(Yeast-like infection causing meningitis and infections in the respiratory tract)

Mycobacterium Avium-Intracellular (MAI) Infection
(TB-like infection in gastrointestinal tract, liver, and bone marrow)

Isosporiasis
(Common cause of diarrhea in AIDS patients)

Herpes Simplex Virus
(Infection of the mouth, esophagus, and lungs)

Candidiasis
(Yeast infections of the mouth, esophagus, trachea, bronchial tubes, and lungs)

Kaposi's Sarcoma

Tuberculosis
(Increased incidence in HIV infected persons)

AIDS Dementia Complex

Lymphoma

Cytomegalovirus
(Infection of the retina and other organs)

1. **AIDS dementia complex** occurs in approximately two-thirds of patients. Confusion, memory loss, and difficulties with concentration are reported symptoms.

2. **Dysarthria** may be present, depending upon the motor and sensory systems involved.

3. In pediatric AIDS cases, high rates of inflammatory ear disease and chronic middle ear effusion that precipitates **hearing impairment** have been identified.

4. Infants with AIDS may fail to develop language and may even remain mute.

D. Pharmacologic Treatment

There are no drugs or vaccines currently available that will prevent or cure HIV infection or AIDS.

1. **Azidothymidine (Zidovudine®) (AZT) (Retrovir®)** is thought to interfere with essential enzyme systems to prevent the growth and reproduction of HIV particles within tissue cells, thus, slowing the progression of HIV infection. AZT is not a cure for ARC or AIDS nor does it provide treatment for opportunistic infections or other complications of HIV infection. AZT does not reduce the risk of transmitting AIDS.

    a. **Desired effects** are a significant delay in the progression of AIDS in HIV infected individuals who are asymptomatic; reduced incidence of infection in persons with ARC and AIDS; and prolongation of life for patients with AIDS.

    > A study of 338 patients with HIV but no evidence of AIDS showed that patients treated early with AZT survived no longer than those treated late. However, the data indicated that early treatment with AZT delayed the development of AIDS from HIV infection.

    b. **Undesirable effects.** Headache, nausea, stomach pain, tremors, and seizures are common. Additional complications are serious anemia and loss of white blood cells (WBCs) and bone marrow depression. An enlarged, fatty liver in HIV infected patients, particularly in obese women, and rare cases of acute hepatitis have been reported.

2. **Didanosine (DDI) (Videx®)** may be recommended for patients who are unresponsive to or intolerant of AZT.

3. **Zalcitabine (dideoxycytidine) (DDC) (Hyvid®)** is an investigational drug that may have a more potent effect than AZT or **DDI**.

4. Several additional drugs are being investigated, but none have proved to prevent or cure AIDS or to protect against the complications of the disease.

5. Table 4–2 lists drugs used to treat opportunistic infections of AIDS, and the side effects of these drugs. Unlike uninfected

TABLE 4–2. Drugs used to treat complications (opportunistic infections) associated with HIV and AIDS.

Opportunistic Infection	Drugs	Side Effects
Pneumocystis carinii pneumonia (PCP)	Trimethoprim	Skin rash, excessive hair growth, tremors, severe kidney injury, hypertension, rare blood cell disorders
	Sulfimethoxazole	Skin rash, headache, dizziness, ataxia, tinnitus, loss of appetite, gastrointestinal disturbance, abdominal pain, painful joints, anaphylaxis, allergic hepatitis, bone marrow depression, fever, pharyngitis, abnormal bleeding or bruising, kidney damage, and peripheral neuropathy
	Pentamidine (Nebupent®)	Skin rash, coughing, wheezing, chest congestion, rare pancreatitis, rare kidney damage
Severe pneumocystis carinii pneumonia (PCP)	Trimetrexate glucuronate (Neutrexin®)	Fewer side effects than other drugs. First drug to be approved for severe PCP.
Toxoplasmosis	Sulfadiazine	Skin rash, swelling of face, redness of eyes, fever, headache, dizziness, ataxia, tinnitus, numbness and tingling in extremities, reduced appetite, mouth irritation, gastrointestinal disturbance, anaphylactic reaction, bone marrow depression, drug-induced hepatitis, drug-induced kidney damage, impaired thyroid function
Mycobacterium avium infections	Clofazimine (Lamperene®)	Skin rash; dry, rough or scaly skin changes; altered taste; loss of appetite; irritation and burning of eyes; severe gastrointestinal disturbance
	Ciprofoxacin (Cipro®)	Skin rash; dizziness, headache, weakness, gastrointestinal disturbance. Rare side effects are restlessness, tremor, confusion, hallucinations, seizures
Herpes Simplex Virus	Acyclovir (Zovirax®)	Skin rash, headache, nervousness, insomnia, depression, fatigue, gastrointestinal disturbance, joint pain, muscle cramping, acne, hair loss, superficial thrombophlebitis, enlarged lymph glands, hallucinations, confusion, paranoia, and depression.

(continued)

TABLE 4–2 (continued). Drugs used to treat complications (opportunistic infections) associated with HIV and AIDS.

Opportunistic Infection	Drugs	Side Effects
Candidiasis	Fluconazole (Diflucan®)	Skin rash, headache, gastrointestinal disturbance, abnormal bleeding or bruising
	Clotrimazole (Lotrimin®)	Skin rash, gastrointestinal disturbance
	Ketoconazole (Nizoral®)	Skin rash, gastrointestinal disturbance, anaphylactic reaction, abnormal bleeding and bruising, altered menstrual patterns
Tuberculosis	Pyrazinamide	Skin rash, fever, loss of appetite, gastrointestinal disturbance, drug-induced hepatitis, gouty arthritis
	Isoniazid (Laniazid®; Teebaconin®)	Skin rash, fever, painful muscles, joint pain, dizziness, gastrointestinal disturbance, peripheral neuritis, acute mental and behavioral disturbances, impaired vision, increased seizure activity, bone marrow depression, fatigue, weakness, pharyngitis, abnormal bleeding or bruising
	Rifampin (Rifamate®)	Discoloration of tears and skin, skin rash, fever, headache, drowsiness, dizziness, blurred vision, impaired hearing, numbness and tingling of extremities, flu-like syndrome, drug-induced liver damage, drug-induced kidney damage, abnormal bleeding or bruising

persons for whom antibiotics can be used to help the body over-come the infectious agent, patients with AIDS are unable to elimi-nate the organisms once the antibiotics have taken effect. For AIDS patients, the antibiotics used for various infections must be contin-ued indefinitely to maintain control of the infectious agent.

E. Effects of the Drugs on Communication Impairment

1. AZT has been reported to have temporary benefit in AIDS demen-tia complex. Drug therapy for opportunistic infections or neo-plasms in the brain may reverse the severity of aphasia, dementia, or dysarthria.

2. Some drugs may have a deleterious affect on communication (*see* Table 4–2.).

3. To date, no drug other than AZT has been reported to have a posi-tive effect on communication impairment.

F. Alternative Treatments

1. Physical therapy may be prescribed for control of weakness and for generalized conditioning.

2. Speech-language therapy may improve communication. Providing the patient and caregiver with strategies for optimum communication may be beneficial.

G. Recommended Readings

Adams, K. M. (1991). The neuropsychology of AIDS. In J. Brooks, (Ed.), Special Interest Division No. 2: *Neurophysiology and Neurogenic Speech and Language Disorders Newsletter.* (Available from American Speech-Language Hearing Association, Rockville, Md.)

Long, J. A. (1993). The essential guide to prescription drugs. New York: Harper Collins.

McGuire, D. (1991). Infectious disease. In M. A. Samuels, (Ed.). *Manual of neurologic therapeutics with essentials of diagnosis* (4th ed.) Boston Toronto; Little, Brown.

Price, R. W. (1988). The brain in AIDS: Central nervous system HIV infection and AIDS dementia complex. *Science, 239,* 586.

Singer, E. J. (1991). Central nervous system (CNS) sequelae of HIV disease. In J. Brooks, (Ed.). Special Interest Division No. 2: *Neurophysiology and Neurogenic Speech and Language Disorders Newsletter, 2* (2). (Available from American Speech-Language Hearing Association, Rockville, MD.)

I. ALZHEIMER'S DISEASE

A. Definition/Cause

1. The exact cause of Alzheimer's disease is unknown. There are changes in the cerebral cortex with widespread loss of neurons. In addition, there is degeneration of the basal nuclei deep within the hemisphere where the neurons use the neurotransmitter acetylcholine and project throughout the cerebral cortex.

2. Approximately one million Americans are diagnosed with Alzheimer's disease each year.

3. The condition is more common in women than in men. Genetic predisposition is highly probable, since Alzheimer's disease occurs is four times more frequently among family members than in the general population.

4. Irregularities of brain that underlie Alzheimer's disease are neurofibrillary tangles, senile neuritic plaques, and granulovacuolar degeneration.

   a. **Neurofibrillary tangles** occur in the cell nucleus as well as near the axons and dendrites. The nucleus becomes filled with a mass of intertwined protein filaments. The presence of neurofibrillary tangles in the frontal and temporal lobes and in the hippocampus is a strong indication of Alzheimer's disease.

   b. **Senile neuritic plaques.** These masses of amyloid protein materials are broken off and they decay healthy nerve endings. The presence of these plaques, in combination with the presence of the neurofibrillary tangles, contributes to the diagnosis of Alzheimer's disease.

   c. Granulovacuolar degeneration. This sign appears when granular materials and fluid-filled vacuoles are seen crowded inside the body of the neuron, particularly in the hippocampus.

In 1906, Dr. Alois Alzheimer discovered the disease that bears his name after studying samples of brain tissue taken from a 55-year-old woman. For some years after this discovery, Alzheimer's disease was assumed to affect only middle-aged patients. All older persons who exhibited Alzheimer's

continued

disease-like behaviors were dismissed as being a little "touched in the head" or "senile." It was not until the 1950s that physicians began to realize that senility was an actual disease that required treatment, plus a great deal of specialized care.

B. General Features, Symptoms, and Signs

1. The onset is insidious. Memory loss is an early feature, and is the hallmark of the disease. Disorientation and confusion occur, and appear to be worse at night than during the day. There is a progressive decline that eventually involves all aspects of cognition.

2. Mood change, apathy, depression, irritability, anxiety, and paranoia are symptoms of the dementia that characterizes Alzheimer's disease.

3. Eventually patients gradually become inactive. Finally, there are gait disturbances and incoordination.

4. Later in the disease process, social skills deteriorate.

5. Most patients die within 4–10 years after diagnosis. The mean duration of survival after diagnosis is 7 years.

C. Features, Symptoms, and Signs of Communication Impairment

1. In the early stages of the disease, patients may exhibit good memory for remote events but begin to show deficits in immediate recall and short-term memory.

2. In the early stages, language may be quite normal, with no impairment of phonology or syntax, but disorientation to time and place begin to occur. Signs of distractibility, memory deficits, and overall intellectual deterioration appear.

3. Soon, thereafter, dementia can be documented from performance on mental status tests and evaluations of cognition and language functions.

4. There is gradual, progressive deterioration of specific cognitive functions such as perception, memory, concentration, and finally a complete loss of the ability to communicate effectively.

D. Pharmacologic Treatment

1. There is loss of acetylcholine in the brain of Alzheimer's patients, and therefore drugs that enhance cholinergic activity in the central nervous system have been investigated for use in Alzheimer's disease. **Tacrine hydrochloride (Cognex®)** is a reversible, centrally acting cholinesterase inhibitor (anticholinesterase) used to attempt to enhance cholinergic activity. This drug is not a cure nor has it been shown to prevent the progression of the disease. In 1993, the Peripheral and Central Nervous System Drugs Advisory Committee to the Food and Drug Administration (FDA) approved tacrine as the first drug designed specifically to treat the symptoms of mild to moderate Alzheimer's disease.

   a. **Desired effects** are cognitive benefits, including improved memory, attention, reasoning, language, and the ability to perform simple tasks.

   b. **Undesirable effects.** The most frequent side effects appear to be **sweating, diarrhea, increased urination, nausea,** and **abdominal discomfort.** Both dose reduction and drugs that inhibit parasympathetic autonomic activity in the GI tract are used to reverse these effects. The most significant side effect has been **liver enzyme irregularities.** Liver enzymes have returned to baseline when the dose was decreased, or the drug was discontinued, but because of this side effect, only slightly more than one-half of patients who were started on tacrine have been able to continue it.

   c. Although some symptomatic improvement has been noted during clinical trials, tacrine's place in therapy for Alzheimer's disease probably needs to be defined with more and longer clinical trials.

E. Effects of the Drug on Communication (See **previous section, Desired Effects**)

F. Alternative Treatments

1. Speech-language therapy may be beneficial in selected cases.

2. Counseling of family members and other caregivers regarding the most effective methods of communication with the patient with Alzheimer's disease is a common procedure.

G. Recommended Readings

Bayles, K., (Ed.). (1992). Human memory and overview. Special Interest Division No. 2 *Neurophysiology and Neurogenic Speech and Language Disorders Newsletter.* (Available from American Speech-Language Hearing Association, Rockville, MD.)

Bourgeois, M.S. (1991). Communication treatment for adults with dementia. *Journal of Speech and Hearing Research, 34,* 831–844.

Carrow, D. L. (1990). *When your loved one has Alzheimer's: A caregiver's guide.* New York: Harper & Row.

Farlow, M., Gracon, S. I., & Hershey, L. A. (1992). A controlled trial of tacrine in Alzheimer's disease. *Journal of the American Medical Association, 268*(18), 2523–2529.

Davis, K. L., Leon, J. T., & Elkan, R. G. (1992). A double-blind, placebo-controlled multicenter study of tacrine for Alzheimer's disease. *New England Journal of Medicine, 327,* 1253-1259.

III. TRAUMATIC BRAIN INJURY (TBI)

A. Definition/Cause

1. In traumatic brain injury, the mechanisms of damage to the brain are several. They include macroscopically visible injury, such as laceration by a penetrating object; hemorrhage into the brain substance; infarction by damage to or compression of cerebral vessels; and hypoxia/hypotension during the acute injury.

2. Even in the absence of these mechanisms, substantial dysfunction may occur after significant head injury. For example, during the sudden acceleration/deceleration with both linear and torsional movement of the brain, individual axons may be stretched and broken so that significant dysfunction occurs without obvious, visible lesions on neuroradiological scans or even evidence in clinical neurologic examination.

3. Most traumatic brain injuries in adults are caused by vehicle and work accidents. In children, most TBIs are caused by accidents at play and by falls.

B. General Features, Symptoms, and Signs

The most common, serious acute problem associated with severe head injury is the elevated level of intracranial pressure (ICP) from cerebral edema, extensive contusions, or hematomas.

C. Features, Symptoms, and Signs of Communication Impairment

Patients with brain injury can display a variety of levels of altered states of consciousness and impaired cognitve functions. Symptoms of traumatic brain injury can include dysarthria as well as language and cognitve disorders.

D. Pharmacologic Treatment

1. The type of medication used depends upon the nature of the injury and the symptoms to be treated. Diuretics, barbiturates, and corticosteroids are used to reduce cerebral edema and ICP.

2. **Diuretics.** Acute elevations of ICP are treated with **mannitol (Osmitrol®).**

   a. **Desired effect** is reduction of ICP.

   b. **Undesirable effects.** Mannitol's effects may reverse within 8-12 hours after administration. Additional, undesirable reactions are **headache, confusion, blurred vision, nausea,** and **cellular dehydration resulting in thirst.**

   c. **Furosemide®,** another diuretic, may be given with mannitol. Possible adverse effects of Furosemide are **dehydration, abdominal pain,** and **skin rash. Transient deafness** can occur if the intravenous injection of Furosemide is too rapid. **Tinnitus, sore throat** and **fever** may be signs of Furosemide toxicity.

3. **Barbiturates. Pentobarbital (Nebralin®, Maso-Pent®, Nembutal®, Nova-Rectal®, Penital®, Pentogen®) and phenobarbital (Luminal®)** are barbiturates given to **induce** coma and thereby reduce metabolic requirements of the brain. Common side effects of barbiturates are **drowsiness, sedation, lethargy, skin rash,** and **nausea.**

4. **Corticosteroids.** The overall effect of steroids on outcome of TBI is not known.

    a. Desired Effect is reduction of focal, cerebral edema.

    b. Undesirable effects. *See* Table 2–3 for side effects of corticosteroids.

5. **Anticonvulsants.** A delayed complication of TBI is seizures. The incidence of posttraumatic epilepsy varies with extent of brain damage, location of the damage (lesions in the area around the Rolandic region are highly likely to produce seizures), and the presence of infection. Seizures are treated with anticonvulsant drugs (*see* Epilepsy for anticonvulsant drugs, and their desired and undesirable effects).

6. Patients who experience headache, dizziness, insomnia, irritability, inability to concentrate, and personality changes have been treated with a variety of drugs, including antidepressants, antipsychotics, and antiparkinson's agents.

E. Effects of the Drugs on Communication

The effects of drugs on communication are varied (*see* sections on Parkinson's disease, epilepsy, depression, anxiety, and schizophrenia, for drugs that may be prescribed for patients with TBI).

F. Alternative Treatments

A variety of alternative treatments, including surgery, physical therapy, speech-language therapy, and patient and family counseling may be necessary for persons who have sustained TBI.

G. Recommended Readings

Carter, J. E., & Vogel, D. (1992). Some drugs used in the treatment of traumatic brain injury. In D. Vogel, (Ed.). Drug Treatment Issues. Special Interest Division 2. *Neurophysiology and Neurogenic Speech and Language Disorders Newsletter,* 2(2), (Available from American Speech-Language-Hearing Association, Rockville, MD.)

Martuza, R. L. & Aquino, T. M. (1986). Trauma: Severe head injury. In M.A. Samuels, (Ed.), *Manual of neurologic therapeutics* (3rd ed., pp. 243–258) Boston/Toronto: Little, Brown.

CHAPTER

5

Psychiatric Disorders

This chapter covers psychiatric disorders that may affect communication. For each disorder, we provide a definition and cause; discuss the general features, symptoms and signs; describe the features, symptoms and signs of communication impairment associated with each disorder; list pharmacologic treatment for each disorder; and discuss the influence drug treatment may have on communication.

I. DEPRESSION

A. Definition/Causes

1. Depression is a disorder that affects mood and cognition. Although the causes of depression are not known, several etiologies have been hypothesized, including dysfunctional family life, psychosocial stress, and neurotransmitter dysfunction. A leading hypothesis is that depression is caused by impaired neurotransmission.

2. A number of medical conditions can cause depression. Some of these conditions are: AIDS, asthma, tuberculosis and other chronic

infections, congestive heart failure, diabetes, Parkinson's disease, malignancies, stroke, multiple sclerosis, rheumatoid arthritis, systemic lupus erythematosis, and malnutrition.

B. General Features, Symptoms, and Signs

Sadness, despair, emptiness; loss of ability to experience pleasure; low self-esteem; apathy; low motivation; social withdrawal; excessive emotional sensitivity; negative, pessimistic thinking; guilt; irritability; suicidal ideation; sleep and appetite disturbances; fatigue; decreased sex drive; restlessness; agitation; psychomotor retardation; and impaired concentration are general features of depression.

C. Features, Symptoms, and Signs of Communication Impairment

Increased latency of responding, decreased length of utterance (sometimes to one word), decreased reliability of information, decreased ability to concentrate, lowered pitch, monopitch, monoloudness (decreased voice volume), and decreased speech rate are features of communication impairment associated with depression.

The author William Styron wrote that the depressed person experiences failure of appetite; failure of forced laughter; and, at last, **virtually total failure of speech.** Styron's own depression was a "ferocious inwardness of pain that produced an immense distraction" preventing his ability to **"articulate words beyond a hoarse murmur."** He sensed himself turning **"wall-eyed and monosyllabic."** "My speech," wrote Styron, "emulating my way of walking, **slowed to the vocal equivalent of a shuffle."** Of the voice change that occurred with his depression, he wrote: "I remember the lamentable **near disappearance of my voice.** It underwent a strange transformation, becoming at times **quite faint, wheezy, and spasmodic.** A friend observed that it was the voice of a 90 year old." (Styron, 1990)

D. Pharmacologic Treatment

1. **Tricyclic antidepressants** are basic in the treatment of depression. For a number of years, tricyclics (so called because they contain

three cyclic rings in their structure) were the major antidepressant medications. These drugs are thought to block serotonin and norepinephrine reuptake. They include **imiprimine hydrochloride (Tofranil®), trimipramine maleate (Surmontil®), amitriptyline (Elavil®), clomipramine hydrochloride (Anafranil®), doxepine hydrochloride (Sinequan®), desipramine (Norpramin®), protriptyline (Vivactil®), and nortriptyline hydrochloride (Pamelor®).**

a. **Desired effect** is relief from the symptoms of depression. The effectiveness in treating depression is similar among these drugs; however, a particular individual may respond well to one antidepressant but not to another.

b. **Undesirable effects.** For many patients, side effects of the tricyclics are minor annoyances, and many side effects will decrease in severity with time. However, some patients may experience **sleep disorders, agitation, confusion, weight gain/loss, gastrointestinal disturbances, tremor, headache, dry mouth, hallucinations, delusions,** and **seizures.**

2. Newer antidepressant drugs contain chemical structures different from that of tricyclics but have similar effectiveness. These antidepressants inhibit serotonin reuptake and include: **fluoxetine hydrochloride (Prozac®), setraline hydrochloride (Zoloft®), trazodone hydrochloride (Desyrel®), bupropion hydrochloride (Welbutrin®), and paroxetine (Paxil®).**

a. **Desired effect.** Relief from depression.

b. **Undesirable effects.** *See* Table 5–1 for the side effects of the newer antidepressant drugs.

Fluoxetine (Prozac®) has received a great deal of attention in both the professional and lay press. It appears that Prozac® may be capable of changing the very identity of a person who takes the drug. For example, it may turn a shy person into an outgoing one. It has been shown that Prozac® has many medical as well as psychiatric side effects. A wide variety of medical, ethical, and moral issues have arisen related to the decision of whether, and for whom, to prescribe this drug.

Table 5–1. Side effects of newer antidepressant drugs.

Drug	Side Effects
Fluoxetine hydrochloride (Prozac®)	Restlessness; insomnia, skin rash, CNS stimulation, anorexia and weight loss, impaired motor performance, anxiety, seizures, tremor, diaphoresis (excessive sweating), gastrointestinal disturbance, precipitation of mania, weakness, dizziness, decreased libido, dry mouth, hypoglycemia, viral infection, fever, congestion, cough, sinusitis, palpitations, back, joint or muscular pain, and visual disturbances
Setraline hydrochloride (Zoloft®)	CNS stimulation, fever, back pain, hot flashes, thirst, weight loss, gastrointestinal disturbance, anxiety, insomnia, dizziness, sexual dysfunction, somnolence, tremor, dry mouth, agitation, skin rash, syncope, chest pain, palpitations, headache
Trazodone hydrochloride (Desyrel®)	Drowsiness, dizziness, fainting, fatigue, CNS stimulation, headache, gastrointestinal disturbance, dry mouth, blurred vision, hypotension, syncope, extrapyramidal symptoms, arrhythmias, leukopenia, seizures, impotence
Bupropion hydrochloride (Wellbutrin®)	CNS stimulation, dry mouth, constipation, agitation, insomnia, headache (including migraine), nausea and vomiting, constipation, weight loss or gain, tremors, seizures (3-4 times more common than with other antidepressants), psychosis
Paroxetine (Paxil®)	Fatigue, somnolence, tremor, dry mouth, constipation, blurred vision, insomnia, decreased libido, dizziness, headache, weight loss or gain, sedation, anxiety, hypotension, rash, sexual dysfunction, asthenia, manic episodes, palpitation, vasodilation, gastrointestinal disturbance.

3. Monoamine Oxidase Inhibitors (MAOIs) increase epinephrine, norepinepherine, and serotonin. The most commonly prescribed MAOIs are **phenelzine (Nardil®), tranylcypromine (Parnate®),** and **isocarboxazid (Marplan®),** These drugs are prescribed for patients who have failed to respond to other antidepressant drugs.

a. **Desired effect** is relief from symptoms of depression.

b. **Undesirable effects.** Certain medications, such as psychostimulants (amphetamines); diet pills and preparations; cold preparations (excluding antihistamines and aspirin, but including over-the counter products which contain decongestants, such as Sudafed® or Contact®) nasal sprays, and adrenaline must be avoided. In addition, a variety of foods must not be eaten by persons taking these drugs. *See* Table 5–2 for a list of foods to avoid while taking MAOIs. Symptoms of drug or food interaction with MAOIs are **severe headache, excessive perspiration, lightheadedness, vomiting,** and **increased heart rate.** A severe side effect is a **sudden and significant increase in blood pressure leading to severe hypertensive crisis.** Symptoms of hypertensive crisis are **headache, diaphoresis, mydriasis, hypertension, neck stiffness, photophobia, tachycardia, bradycardia, angina, nausea,** and **vomiting.**

Table 5–2. Foods and drugs to avoid while taking MAO inhibitors.

Fruits: Canned figs, raisins, bananas, overripe fruit

Vegetables: Fava beans (Italian green beans), sauerkraut, avocados, bean curd, soy sauce

Dairy: Aged yogurt, strong cheeses, sour cream

Meat: Liver (chicken and beef), fermented sausages (bologna, salami, pepperoni), meat tenderizer, meat extracts

Fish: Dried salted fish, pickled or dried (kippered) herring, caviar, shrimp paste

Beverages: Beer, Chianti and other red wines, sherry, non-distilled alcohol

Other foods: Yeast, caffeine, protein extracts (found in some dried soups; soup cubes, and commercial gravies)

Drugs: Stimulant drugs (*see* Attention Deficit Hyperactivity Disorder), diet pills, cocaine, "crack," cold preparations, including decongestants and nasal sprays, adrenaline (found in many local anesthetics)

c. **Lithium carbonate (Lithobid®)** is used primarily in the treatment of manic-depressive illness but also may be used when depression occurs alone (*see* Manic-Depressive Illness for desired and undesirable effects of lithium carbonate).

4. **Investigational Drugs**

a. **Doathiepin hydrochloride (Prothiaden®)** is a drug that has not yet been approved for use in the United States. It appears to be comparable to other tricyclic antidepressants in the treatment of depression.
   (1) **Desired effect.** Treatment of depression with a low incidence of anticholinergic side effects (*see* Glossary).
   (2) **Undesirable effects** are drowsiness, dry mouth, gastrointestinal disturbances, tremor, dizziness, sweating, insomnia, weight gain, blurred vision, palpitations, and headache.

b. **Fluvoxamine (Floxfral®).** This drug appears to be useful in patients who are unable to tolerate tricyclic antidepressants.
   (1) **Desired effect** is treatment of depression.
   (2) **Undesirable effects** are **nausea and vomiting, constipation, headache, dry mouth, agitation, somnolence, tremor, agitation, dizziness, syncope, manic episodes, insomnia,** and **anorexia.**

E. Effects of the Drugs on Communication

When effective, antidepressant drugs will control or eliminate the symptoms and signs of depression and, therefore, the symptoms and signs of communication impairment associated with the depression.

F. Alternative Treatments

1. **Psychotherapy** has been beneficial either as the primary therapy or in conjunction with antidepressant drugs.

2. **Electroconvulsive therapy (ECT)** produces seizures presumably to bring about change in neurotransmitter function. The induction of bilateral generalized seizures is necessary for the beneficial effects of ECT. The response rate to ECT for patients with major depression is 80–90%, which is at least equal to the response rate to antidepressant drugs.

a. The symptoms of severe psychomotor retardation, sleep distur-bance, decreased appetite and weight loss, and agitation are most likely to respond to ECT.

b. An undesirable effect of ECT is memory impairment that may occur during the course of the treatment. Although follow-up studies have indicated that, for most patients, memory returns to baseline condition after 6 months, the degree of cognitive impairment during treatment and the time it takes to return to baseline is related, in part, to the amount of electrical stimula-tion that was used during the ECT sessions.

3. **Psychosurgery.** If severe depression persists for 3 years or more and if alternative treatment approaches are unsuccessful, modifying the brain surgically to reduce symptoms may be considered. The interest in psychosurgery that waned after psychotropic drugs were introduced is being discussed currently and is considered by some professionals as a possible alternative treatment.

G. Recommended Readings

Arana, G. W. & Hyman, S. E. (1991). *Handbook of psychiatric drug therapy* (2nd ed.). Boston: Little, Brown.

Burwell, L. (1994). Handbook of psychiatric drugs. *Current clinical strategies* (3rd ed.). Philadelphia: W. B. Saunders.

Jones, J. M., & Schamburg, R. (1991). *Everything you need to know about Prozac.* New York: Bantam Books.

Kramer, P. D. (1993). *Listening to Prozac.* New York: Viking Press.

Preston, J., & Johnson, J. (1991). *Clinical psychopharmacology made ridicu-lously simple.* Miami, FL: MedMaster, Inc.

Styron, W. (1990). *Darkness visible: A memoir of madness.* New York: Random House.

II. MANIA

A. Definition/Cause

The person in a manic state is cheerful, talkative, and grandiose; has ele-vated self-esteem; is hyperenergetic, hypersexual; and exhibits a decreased need for sleep.

B. General Features, Symptoms, and Signs

Signs of mania are manifested in poor judgment and lack of resistance. For example, the patient may engage in buying sprees, compulsive gambling, or give away money.

C. Features, Symptoms, and Signs of Communication Impairment

Rapid, pressured speech that is often impossible to interrupt, incomplete sentences, and labile pitch are features of communication impairment. The patient often is described as exhibiting a "flight of ideas" or a rapid switching of topics.

D. Pharmacologic Treatment

Mood stabilizers are lithium carbonate (Lithobid®), carbamazepine (Tegretol®), and valproic acid (Depakote®).

1. Lithium carbonate (Lithobid®)

   a. **Desired effect** is reduction of the manic episode.

   b. **Undesirable effects.** Side effects of lithium are **gastrointestinal disturbance, fine tremor in the hand, sedation, muscular weakness, polyuria (frequent urination), polydypsia (frequent thirst), edema, weight gain,** and **dry mouth.** More severe side effects are **increase in white blood cells** and **kidney damage.**

   Signs of lithium toxicity are **lethargy, ataxia, arrhythmia, hypotension, seizures, shock delirium, coma,** and **death.**

2. Carbamazepine (Tegretol®)

   a. **Desired effect** is treatment of acute mania.

   b. **Undesirable effects. Bone marrow depression** or **elevated liver enzymes** may occur early in the use of Tegretol. **Skin rash, headache, dizziness or vertigo, drowsiness, ataxia, fatigue, blurred vision, confusion, tinnitus, loss of appetite, gastrointestinal disorders, edema, changes in skin pigmentation, hair loss, aching of muscles,** and **joint and leg cramps** are all milder side effects of carbamazepine. Serious adverse effects include **severe dermatitis,** with **irritation of mouth and**

tongue; swelling of lymph glands; kidney damage; depression and agitation; diplopia; visual hallucinations; peripheral neuritis; and **thrombophlebitis. Latent psychosis and systemic lupus erythematosus** may be activated by this drug.

3. Valproic acid (Depakene®) (Depakote®)

   a. Desired effect is control of symptoms of bipolar disorder.

   b. Undesirable effects. Valproic acid produces **central nervous
system depression, elevations of liver enzymes and hepatitis, gastrointestinal disturbance, drowsiness, ataxia,
headache,** and **skin rash. Substantial weight gain** is a common problem.

E. Effects of the Drugs on Communication Impairment

1. Lithium controls the symptoms of mania and therefore, the rapid
speech and flight of ideas that are features of the communication
impairment associated with mania.

2. Signs of lithium toxicity affecting communication are **dysarthria,
tinnitus,** and **oral-facial tremor.**

F. Alternative Treatments

Psychotherapy is an important component of treatment for mania.

G. Recommended Readings

Preston, J., & Johnson, J. (1991). C*linical pyschopharmacology made ridicu-
lously simple.* Miami, FL: MedMaster, Inc.
Burwell, L. (1994). *Handbook of psychiatric drugs: Current clinical strategies.*
Fountain Valley, CA: Current Clinical Strategies Publishing.

III. MANIC-DEPRESSIVE ILLNESS (BIPOLAR DISORDER)

A. Description/Cause

1. Bipolar disorder is a recurring illness in which mania, characterized
by elevated, expansive, or irritable mood, alternates with symptoms
of depression.

2. Manic patients often drink alcohol excessively, are disinhibited,
and may be impulsive.

   3. In approximately 50% of bipolar patients, there is a family history of the illness.

B. General Features, Symptoms, and Signs

   1. Episodes of mania, depression, or a combination of the two are characteristic of bipolar illness. Typically, there is rapid onset of the manic episode but these episodes can evolve over days or weeks.

   2. The manic episode cycles into an episode of depression.

C. Features, Symptoms, and Signs of Communication Impairment

   See Depression and Mania.

D. Pharmacologic Treatments

   1. Lithium carbonate

   a. Desired effects. Reduction of the manic and depressive episodes.

   b. Undesirable Effects. Side effects of lithium are gastrointestinal **disturbance, fine tremor of the hand, sedation, muscular weakness, polyuria (frequent urination), polydypsia (frequent thirst), edema, weight gain,** and **dry mouth.**

   More severe side effects are **increase in white blood cells and kidney damage.** Signs of **lithium toxicity** are **lethargy, ataxia, arrhythmia, hypotension, seizures, shock, delirium, coma,** and **death.**

E. Effects of the Drug on Communication Impairment

   1. Lithium controls the symptoms of mania and therefore, the rapid speech and flight of ideas that are features of the communication impairment.

   2. Signs of lithium toxicity affecting communication are dysarthria, tinnitus, and oral-facial tremor.

F. Alternative Treatment

   Psychotherapy is an important component of treatment for bipolar illness.

IV. ANXIETY DISORDER

A. Definition/Cause

1. Although it is not possible to identify every cause of anxiety, some causes have been noted.

2. Some medical conditions commonly associated with anxiety are CNS degenerative disease, Cushing's syndrome (*see* Glossary), coronary insufficiency, hypoglycemia, hyperthyroidism, early stages of Meniere's disease, postconcussion syndrome, PMS, and mitral valve prolapse.

3. Some drugs that can cause anxiety are amphetamines, corticosteroids, caffeine, asthma medications, nasal decongestant sprays, and cocaine.

B. General Features, Symptoms, and Signs

Trembling, muscle tension, shortness of breath, a smothering sensation, tachycardia, sweating, cold hands and feet, lightheadedness and dizziness, paresthesia, diarrhea and/or frequent urination, feelings of unreality, sleep alteration, nervousness and irritability, and akathisia (*see* Glossary), are all symptoms and signs of anxiety disorder.

C. Features, Symptoms, and Signs of Communication Impairment

Impaired attention and concentration are symptoms of anxiety that affect communication.

D. Pharmacologic Treatment (Anxiolytics)

1. **Benzodiazepines** are drugs used to treat symptoms of anxiety. These drugs seem to potentiate GABA (*see* Chapter 1). Commonly prescribed benzodiazepines include **alprazolam (Xanax®), chlordiazepoxide hydrochloride (Librium®), clorazepate dipotassium (Tranxene®), diazepam (Valium®), halezepam (Paxipam®), flurazepam hydrochloride (Dalmane®), lorazepam (Ativan®), oxazepam (Serax®), Prazepam (Centrax®), estazolam (ProSom®), quazepam (Doral®), clonazepam (Klonipin®), temazepam (Restoril®), and triazolam (Halcion®).** Table 5–3 lists the most common side effects of benzodiazepines.

Elderly persons will require smaller doses of benzodiazepines over longer intervals to avoid overdose. **Lethargy, indifference, fatigue, weakness, ataxia, nightmares, paradoxical reactions of excitement, agitation, anger, hostility,** and **rage** are signs of overdose.

2. **Sedatives** used to treat symptoms of anxiety are **meprobamate (Equanil®, Miltown®), hydroxyzine hydrochloride (Atarax®)/ hydroxyzine pamoate (Vistaril®).**

a. **Meprobamate (Equanil®, Miltown®)** acts on the central nervous system and inhibits spinal reflexes.
(1) **Desired effect** is reduction of the symptoms of anxiety.
(2) **Undesirable effects** are **drowsiness, vertigo, CNS depression, weakness, paradoxical excitement, ataxia, gastrointestinal disturbance, allergic reactions, dependence, hypotension, airway obstruction,** and **respiratory depression. Overdose** of this drug is extremely dangerous.

b. **Hydroxyzine hydrochloride (Atarax®)/hydroxyzine pamoate (Vistaril®)** reduces subcortical activity, and also produces muscle relaxant effects.
(1) **Desired effect** is reduction of anxiety.
(2) **Undesirable effects** are **dry mouth, drowsiness, tremor, convulsions,** and **hypersensitivy reactions.** Overdose can cause **CNS depression** and **sedation.**

E. Effects of the Drugs on Communication

1. A number of benzodiazepines cause impaired concentration and memory (*see* Table 5–3).

2. Sedatives used for symptoms of anxiety can cause dysarthria.

F. Alternative Treatments

In general, psychotherapy is recommended in conjunction with drug therapy.

G. Recommended Readings

Abramowicz, M. (1993). Drugs that cause psychiatric symptoms. *The medical letter on drugs and therapeutics.* New York: The Medical Letter, Inc.

Cassena, N. H. *Massachusetts General Hospital's Handbook of General Hospital Psychiatry* (3rd ed.). St. Louis, MO:Mosby.

Kaplan, H. I., & Sadoch, B. J., (1991). *Synopsis of psychiatry* (5th ed.). Baltimore: Williams & Wilkins.

Smith, E., & Faber, R. (1992). Effects of psychotropic medications on speech and language. In D. Vogel, (Ed.). Drug Treatment Issues. Special Interest Division 2. *Neurophysiology and Neurogenic Speech and Language Disorders Newsletter.* 2(2). (Available from American Speech-Language-Hearing Association, Rockville, MD.)

Snyder, S. H. (1988). Psychological disorders and their treatment. *Encyclopedia of health.* New York: Chelsea House Publishers.

Table 5–3. Side effects of commonly used benzodiazepines.

Drug	Side Effects
Alprazolam (Xanax®)	Sedation, CNS depression, impaired concentration and memory, ataxia, drowsiness, hypotension, headache, paradoxical agitation, nausea, vertigo, seizures, tremors
Chlordiazepoxide hydrochloride (Librium®)	Sedation, impaired concentration, ataxia, extrapyramidal effects, drowsiness, hypotension, paradoxical agitation, tolerance and dependence, memory impairments, jaundice, skin rash, edema, decrease in effects of levodopa
Clorazepate dipotassium (Tranxene®)	Sedation, impaired concentration, ataxia, drowsiness, skin rash, headache, hypotension, tolerance and dependence, CNS depression, memory impairment, gastrointestinal disturbance, blurred vision, dry mouth, tremor, abnormal kidney and liver function studies
Diazepam (Valium®)	Sedation, impaired concentration and memory, ataxia, drowsiness, hypotension, nausea
Halazepam (Paxipam®)	Sedation, impaired concentration, ataxia, drowsiness, tolerance, skin rash, hypotension, paradoxical agitation, nausea, vertigo
Flurazepam hydrochloride (Dalmane®)	Elevations of liver function studies, sedation, impaired concentration, blurred vision, ataxia, drowsiness, hypotension, paradoxical agitation, gastrointestinal disturbance, vertigo, tolerance and dependence, headache, lethargy, blood dyscrasias (see Glossary)
Lorazepam (Ativan®)	Impaired concentration and memory, ataxia, hypotension, paradoxical agitation, sedation, nausea, vertigo, tolerance and dependence, headache, dizziness, blood dyscrasias
Oxazepam (Serax®)	Sedation, impaired concentration and memory, ataxia, hypotension, paradoxical agitation, nausea, vertigo, skin rash, tolerance and dependence, dysarthria, dizziness
Prazepam (Cenetrax®)	Sedation, CNS depression, dry mouth, diaphoresis, dysarthria, headache, impaired concentration and memory, ataxia, hypotension, paradoxical agitation, nausea, vertigo, tolerance and dependence

(continued)

Table 5–3. *(continued)*

Estazolam (ProSom®)	Respiratory depression, sedation, CNS depression, impaired concentration, ataxia, hypotension, paradoxical agitation, nausea, vertigo, tolerance, and dependence
Quazepam (Doral®)	Sedation, CNS depression, dry mouth, headache, impaired concentration, ataxia, hypotension, paradoxical agitation, gastrointestinal disturbance, vertigo, tolerance, and dependence
Temazepam (Restoril®)	Sedation, CNS depression, impaired concentration, ataxia, drowsiness, hypotension, paradoxical agitation, gastrointestinal disturbance, anorexia, vertigo, early morning awakening
Triazolam (Halcion®)	Sedation, CNS depression, impaired concentration and memory, ataxia, headache, drowsiness, hypotension, agitation, nausea, and vertigo

V. SCHIZOPHRENIA

A. Definition/Cause

1. Schizophrenia is a group of disorders manifested by severe disturbances of thinking and personality. Although the fundamental cause of schizophrenia is unknown, it is thought to involve the excessive action of dopamine or related neurotransmitters. A genetic predisposition has been suggested as has an environmental etiology.

2. Approximately 1% of the United States population has been diagnosed with schizophrenia. Onset is most common between 16–25 years of age, is uncommon after 30, and is rare after age 40. Incidence is about equal for males and females. Schizophrenia has been described in all cultures and all socioeconomic classes.

3. Some studies have revealed enlarged ventricles in patients with schizophrenia; others have reported no significant difference in ventricle size between schizophrenic and nonschizophrenic sub-

jects. Other studies have shown that brains of persons with schizophrenia weigh less than the brains of nonschizophrenic persons. Several investigators have concluded that persons with schizophrenia have smaller brain structures, such as the limbic system, or cerebellar vermi. Recent PET studies have shown that the most frequent deficits of attention manifested in schizophrenia were in the basal ganglia (globus pallidus) and frontal areas.

B. General Features, Symptoms, and Signs

There is no laboratory test to identify schizophrenia. The CT scans of a large group of schizophrenic patients have revealed enlargement of the lateral and third ventricles as well as cortical atrophy.

1. Although no one symptom or sign is found in all schizophrenic patients, the **most common symptoms** are:

   a. **Alteration of the senses** in which all sensations may be increased. Noises, particularly background noises, may seem louder; colors may appear brighter and detail may be accentuated. A **"flooding" of sensations** may occur in which the ability to screen out incoming stimuli and thus to select the stimulus to which to attend is compromised.

   b. **Flooding of the mind** with thoughts and memories resulting in poor concentration and increased distraction.

   c. **Blunting of sensations,** such as pain, is a possible symptom.

   d. **Thought disorder,** defined as an impairment of the ability to think and express oneself logically, has been identified.

   e. **Changes in emotions (affect).** Early in the illness, the patient may feel **varying and rapidly fluctuating emotions** and, later, may experience exaggerated feelings, guilt, and fear without specific cause. Inappropriate emotions produce one of the most dramatic aspects of schizophrenia. For example, the patient may laugh loudly for no apparent reason or at an inappropriate time, for example, at a funeral.

Flattening (blunting) of emotions reflecting impairment in the ability to empathize with other persons may be subtle in the early stages, but as the disease progresses, becomes more prominent.

---

f. **Changes in movements.** Schizophrenia can cause changes in movements that, in some cases, increase in speed and, in other cases, become slower. **Ataxia and decreased spontaneous arm swing** have been observed. **Tics and tremors** that are not due to medication, but, rather, to the disease process have been observed.

The most dramatic change of movement is **catatonic** behavior during which patients may remain motionless for a long period of time. Catatonia is a symptom that has become much less common with the increased availability of antipsychotic drugs (*see* Pharmacologic Treatment).

g. **Changes in behavior.** Withdrawal with immobility and mutism are common behaviors associated with schizophrenia. Repetitive behaviors such as walking in circles or marching three steps backward and three steps forward are signs, as are ritualistic behaviors such as avoiding stepping on cracks in the sidewalk. Schizophrenic behavior is considered inappropriate to the observer, but to the patient it is always logical and rational.

h. **Delusions** are defined as false ideas, believed by the patient but not by others, that cannot be corrected by reason. Delusions are one of the most common symptoms of schizophrenia. The patient may believe that random events are related to him or her in a direct way. For example, if someone in the room coughs, the person with schizophrenia may be convinced that the cough was meant in some way to convey a message relevant to him or her. Moreover, the patient may be convinced that he or she is being controlled by other persons or things or that he or she is controlling outside events, for example, causing the sun to rise. Attempts to reason schizophrenic patients out of their delusions are rarely successful.

i. **Hallucinations**, gross distortions of sensory stimuli, are common symptoms of schizophrenia. Auditory hallucinations are the most common and may be heard as a single voice, multiple voices, or even choirs of voices heard continually or only occasionally. In a majority of cases the voices are unpleasant, often accusing or blaming the person with schizophrenia for past misdeeds that are either real or imagined.

   (1) The precise mechanism of **auditory hallucinations** is not well understood. The most plausible explanation is that the disease affects the auditory tracts or auditory centers adjacent to the limbic system. It has been reported that individ-

uals who are deaf at birth and who later develop schizophrenia can experience auditory hallucinations.

(2) **Visual hallucinations** are reported less frequently than auditory hallucinations, but, when present, they appear in conjunction with auditory hallucinations. When visual hallucinations appear in isolation, probably schizophrenia is not the cause.

(3) **Hallucinations of touch, smell, and taste** are even less common than visual hallucinations in schizophrenia.

j. **Altered sense of self.** Schizophrenic patients may perceive their body parts to be dissociated and detached and may be unable to distinguish their own bodies from those of other persons or objects. The origin of altered sense of self is unknown, but it is likely that the same disease process responsible for altering senses and thought processes also alters the sense of self.

C. Features, Symptoms, and Signs of Communication Impairment

Perseveration and repetition in verbal, gestural, and graphic responses have been described. Schizophrenic language contains bizarre content replete with neologisms. Additional signs of communication impairment in schizophrenia are listed in Table 5–4.

Neologisms occur in the language of both the aphasic and the schizophrenic patient. It has been suggested that the difference between the use of neologisms in aphasic versus schizophrenic populations is that the aphasic person **wants** the listener to understand whereas the schizophrenic person **doesn't care** whether the listener understands.

D. Pharmacologic Treatment

1. Management of schizophrenia is based on antipsychotic drugs (neuroleptics). When effective, these drugs block dopamine receptors and decrease the symptoms of schizophrenia. Table 5–5 contains a list of the side effects of antipsychotic drugs.

2. **Desired effects.** Drug therapy can abolish delusions, hallucinations, and other bizarre thinking and behavior.

Table 5–4. Features, symptoms, and signs of communication impairment in schizophrenia.

Echolalia

Distractibility

Disruption of auditory processing and retention

Concreteness: Difficulty dealing with abstract concepts with no understanding of nuances of meaning

Limited understanding or use of metaphor

Derailment: Reduction of ability to maintain a "train of thought"

Poverty of speech: Decrease in the amount of speech used. Often limited to monosyllabic replies

Poverty of content of speech: Vague, obscure speech containing little information

Dysprosody and circumlocution

Blocking: Abrupt interruptions after which the speaker has no recall of what was said or what should be said next

Clang associations: Use of words that have no logical association. Words may be similar in sound but not in meaning

Word salad: Incoherent mixture of words and phases

Unintelligible, incomprehensible speech

Mutism

Table 5–5. Desired and undesirable effects of antipsychotic drugs.

Drug	Desired Effect	Undesirable Effects
Haloperidol (Haldol®)/Haloperidol decanoate/Haloperidol lactate	Control of symptoms with lower incidence of sedation and hypotension than other neuroleptics	Sedation, amenorrhea, weight gain, urinary retention, constipation, blurred vision, hypotension, dystonic reactions, akinesia, tardive dyskinesia, Parkinsonism, reduced libido, skin rash, ECG changes, lowered seizure threshold, neuroleptic malignant syndrome

(continued)

Table 5–5. *(continued)*

Drug	Desired Effect	Undesirable Effects
Clozapine (Clozaril®)	Control of symptoms without extrapyramidal side effects. Positive response in patients for whom other neuroleptics are not effective.	Dizziness, seizures, orthostatic hypotension, sedation, gastrointestinal disturbance, fever, anticholinergic effects, cognitive impairment, hypersalivation, tachycardia, EEG and ECG changes, agranulocytosis, granulocytopenia, leukopenia, increase in REM sleep, headache, tremor, restlessness, and agitation.
Loxapine hydrochloride/Locapine succinate (Loxitane®, Daxolin®)	Control of symptoms	Sedation, constipation, dry mouth, blurred vision, hypotension, reduced libido, weight gain, skin rash, photosensitivity, parkinsonism, dystonic reactions, akinesia, tardive dyskinesia, lowered seizure threshold, mania
Molindrone (Moban®)	Control of symptoms Less likely to cause weight gain or impotence than other neuroleptics	Sedation, constipation, blurred vision, reduced libido, skin rash, dry mouth, dystonia, hyperactivity, akinesia, parkinsonism, lowered seizure threshold, neuroleptic malignant syndrome, tardive dyskinesia
Chlorpromazine hydrochloride (Thorazine®)	Control of symptoms	More likely to cause anticholinergic side effects, agranulocytosis, and allergic reactions than other neuroleptics. Hypotension, sedation, constipation, skin

(continued)

Table 5–5. *(continued)*

Drug	Desired Effect	Undesirable Effects
		rash, blurred vision, weight gain dystonia, akinesia, lowered seizure threshold, tardive dyskinesia, parkinsonism, agranulocytosis, neuroleptic malignant syndrome
Promazine hydrochloride (Sparine®)	Control of symptoms	More likely to cause seizures than other neuroleptics. Sedation, dystonia, akinesia, tardive dyskinesia, hypotension, neuroleptic malignant syndrome, weight gain, agranulocytosis, reduced libido, allergic reactions in persons with asthma
Triflupromazine (Vesprin®)	Control of symptoms	Sedation, anticholinergic effects, hypotension, extrapyramidal effects
Thioridazine hydrochloride (Mellaril®)	Control of symptoms with less risk of NMS and extrapyramidal effects than some other neuroleptics	Sexual dysfunction, sedation, constipation, blurred vision, weight gain, skin rash, seizures, dystonia, akinesia, neuroleptic malignant syndrome, retinopathy, jaundice.
Fluphenazine hydrochloride (Prolixin®)	Control of symptoms with less likelihood of causing seizures than other neuroleptics	Sedation, dystonia, akinesia, constipation, skin rash, blurred vision, weight gain, reduced libido, parkinsonism, retinopathy, tardive dyskinesia, neuroleptic malignant syndrome, hypertension, insomnia, jaundice

(continued)

Table 5–5.   *(continued)*

Drug	Desired Effect	Undesirable Effects
Perphenazine (Trilafon®)	Control of symptoms with less likelihood of causing seizures and hypotension than other neuroleptics	Anticholinergic and extrapyramidal side effects. May cause asthma attacks and allergic reactions. Constipation, blurred vision, photosensitivity, hypotension, sedation, dystonia, akinesia, parkinsonism, skin rash, weight gain, jaundice, blood dyscrasias, hyperthermia, retinopathy, tardive dyskinesia, neuroleptic malignant syndrome
Trifluoperazine hydrochloride (Stelazine®)	Control of symptoms with less likelihood of cardiac conduction changes than with other neuroleptics	Constipation, skin rash, blurred vision, weight gain, photosensitivity, sedation, reduced libido, extrapyramidal effects, hypotension, seizures, NMS, tardive dyskinesia, jaundice, retinopathy
Prochlorperazine (Compazine®)	Control of symptoms with less likelihood of seizures than with other neuroleptics	Sedation, constipation, skin rash, blurred vision, dry mouth, salivation, hypotension, weight gain, reduced libido, extrapyramidal effects, neuroleptic malignant syndrome

3. **Undesirable effects.** (*See* Table 5–5.) Extrapyramidal side effects of antipsychotic drugs include:

   a. **Parkinsonism.** Antipsychotic drugs control the symptoms of schizophrenia by blocking dopamine action in the mesolimbic system. Unfortunately, because the drugs also block dopamine action in the nigrostriatal system, they can cause parkinsonism. Drug-induced parkinsonism occurs in 90% of cases within the first 72 days of treatment with a peak onset of 5–30 days. The result is overall **muscular rigidity, resting and intention tremor, pill rolling tremor of the hands, slowed movements or immobility, shuffling gait, cogwheel rigidity, masked facies, dysarthria,** and **dysphagia.**

b. **Tardive dyskinesia** usually is a consequence of long-term antipsychotic drug therapy. Symptoms include **involuntary, bizarre movements of the eyelids, jaws, lips, tongue, neck, and fingers,** and **uncontrollable chewing, lip puckering,** and **repetitive tongue protrusion.**

E. Effects of the Drugs on Communication

1. The tardive dyskinesia resulting from antipsychotic drug use has deleterious effects on communication including general overall, intermittent breakdown in respiration, phonation, articulation, and prosody. Specifically, respiratory dyskinesia occurs with irregular respiration at rest and occasional gasps (audible inspiration), and involuntary vocalizations accompanied by choreic trunk movements, articulatory impairment, and decreased speech fluency.

   a. To date, there is no way to predict who may develop this severe side effect of antipsychotic drugs.

   b. Recently, it has been suggested that **Vitamin E** may alleviate symptoms of tardive dyskinesia.

   c. Tardive dyskinesia may disappear after withdrawal of the antipsychotic medication but, often, it persists. A treatment challenge is to find a balance between the dosage that controls the symptoms of schizophrenia while minimizing the possibility of the occurrence of tardive dyskinesia.

2. **Akathisia** (uncontrolled restlessness) is most common in patients over 30 years of age. Agitation, anxiety, and muscular tremor interfere with communication.

3. **Dystonia**, with muscle spasm and prolonged muscular contractions (usually of the head and neck) with onset of rigidity and cramping, is most likely to occur within the first week of treatment. Frequently it involves the jaw muscles.

4. **Neuroleptic Malignant Syndrome** (NMS) is characterized by unstable body temperature and blood pressure, muscular rigidity,

dysphagia, and mutism. Rapid heart rate and breathing, profuse sweating, tremors, and seizures may be noted. NMS usually occurs within the first week of treatment, but it may occur after hours or after months of treatment. Though rare, this condition is a potentially fatal side effect of antipsychotic drugs (*see* Table 5–5).

F. Alternative Treatments

1. **Psychotherapy** combined with antipsychotic drugs appears to be more effective than medication alone in reducing the number of hospitalizations for patients with schizophrenia. Supportive therapies emphasize providing structure to the patient's life and may help patients distinguish reality from fantasy, learn or relearn social skills, and may educate the patient about the illness. Often, treatment is conducted as group psychotherapy.

2. **Family counseling**. Family members are definite victims of schizophrenia. The illness affects the entire family emotionally and financially. About two thirds of hospitalized schizophrenic patients are discharged to live with family members, usually parents. Others live near their families. Family support groups offer a chance to discuss problems in common, become aware of community resources, and interact with those who are undergoing similar experiences.

G. Recommended Readings

Adler, A. A., Peselow, E., Rotrosin, J., Duncan, E., Lee, M., Rosenthal, M. & Angrist, B. (1993). Vitamin E treatment of tardive dyskinesia. *American Journal of Psychiatry, 150*, 1405–1407.

Calaguiri, M. P., Lohr, J. G., & Jeste, D. V. (1993). Parkinsonism in neuroleptic-naive schizophrenic patients. *American Journal of Psychiatry, 150*, 1343–1348.

DiSimoni, F., Darley, F. L., & Aronson, A. E. (1977). Patterns of dysfunction in schizophrenic patients on an aphasia test battery. *Journal of Speech and Hearing Disorders, 42*, 498–513.

Egan, M. F., Hyde, T. M., Albers, A. E., Alexander, M. D., Reeve, A., Blum, A., Saenz, R. E., & Wyatt, R. J. (1992). Treatment of tardive dyskinesia with vitamin E. *American Journal of Psychiatry, 149*(6), 773–777.

Gerratt, B. R., Goetz, G., & Fisher, H. B. (1984). Speech abnormalities in tardive dyskinesia. *Archives of Neurology, 41*, 273–276.

Kahn, R., Jampala, V. C., Dong, K., & Vedak, C. S. (1994). Speech abnormalities in tardive dyskinesia. *American Journal of Psychiatry, 151*(5), 760–762.

Kane, J. M. (1993). Newer antipsychotic drugs: a review of their pharmacology and therapeutic potential. *Drugs, 46*, 585–593.

Kaplan, B. (1964). *The inner world of mental illness*, New York: Harper & Row.

Kaplan, H. E. & Sadoch, B. J. (1991). *Synopsis of psychiatry* (5th ed.). Baltimore: Williams and Wilkins.

Snyder, S. H. (1990). *Psychological disorders and their treatment: Encyclopedia of health*. New York: Chelsea House Publishers.

Torrey, E. F. (1988). *Surviving schizophrenia. A family manual*. New York: Harper & Row.

Vogel, D., & Rubin, S. (1993, November). Psychiatry, prescription drugs and communication impairment. Miniseminar presented to the American Speech-Language-Hearing Association Convention, Anaheim, CA.

VI. AUTISM

A. Definition/Cause

1. For many years, autism was thought to be a psychological disorder with no organic basis. The cause was explained as a lack of maternal bonding and an experience of rejection that made the infant withdraw into a world of fantasy that the outside world could not penetrate.

2. The rejection theories were not supported by empirical evidence. Therefore, biological causes were considered, for example, **genetic conditions**, such as phenylketonuria, neurofibromatosis, or fragile X syndrome; **viral infections**, such as rubella or herpes encephalitis, and **complications of pregnancy and birth**.

> Post mortem studies have revealed abnormalities in the frontal lobes, limbic system, brain stem, fourth ventricle, or cerebellum. No single defective brain structure has been identified as a contributory cause.

3. Another theory is that persons with autism have a faulty cognitive mechanism that preventing them from engaging in imaginative ideas, interpreting feelings, and understanding intentions beyond the literal content of speech.

B. General Features, Symptoms, and Signs

1. Marked lack of awareness of the existence of feelings of others, no or abnormal seeking of comfort at times of distress, and no or abnormal social play are characteristics of autism. *See* Table 5–6 for a more complete list of features, symptoms, and signs.

Table 5-6. Features, symptoms, and signs of autism.

Marked lack of awareness of the existence of feelings of others

No or abnormal seeking of comfort at times of distress

No or abnormal social play

Gross impairment in ability to establish peer friendships

Stereotyped body movements (hand flicking, head banging)

Persistent preoccupation with parts of objects

Marked distress over changes in trivial aspects of environment

Unreasonable insistence on following routines in precise details

Markedly restricted range of interests, preoccupation with one narrow interest

C. Features, Symptoms, and Signs of Communication Impairment

Impaired or no imitation and an inability to access a mode of communication, such as communicative babbling, facial expression, gesture, mime, or spoken language, are characteristics of autism. Additional features include markedly abnormal nonverbal communication; marked abnormalities in the production of speech, including volume, pitch, stress, rate, rhythm, and intonation; marked abnormalities in the form and content of speech; echolalia, impersonal language, for example, use of "You" when "I" is meant; idiosyncratic use of words or frequent irrelevant remarks; and marked impairment in the ability to initiate or sustain a conversation despite adequate speech.

D. Pharmacologic Treatment

1. Although there is no drug that cures autism, several agents have been investigated. **Fenfluramine** reduces the blood level of serotonin, a neurotransmitter that has been found to be abundant in some children with autism.

2. **Megavitamins**. High doses of vitamin B6 and magnesium have been suggested as treatment for autism. After withdrawal of the treatment, some persons with autism have demonstrated increased symptoms, leading some investigators to believe in the effectiveness of this type of treatment.

3. **Antipsychotics (neuroleptics)** have provided temporary relief from agitation, aggression, insomnia, and repetitive behaviors that may be experienced by persons with autism. Because of the dangerous side effects associated with long-term use (*see* Schizophrenia), these drugs are used only for short-term relief of symptoms.

4. **Naltrexone** is an opiate antagonist, that blocks naturally occurring opioids in the brain. At present this agent is being evaluated for its effectiveness in the treatment of autism and is considered an experimental drug.

E. Effects of Drugs on Communication

1. There is no drug that permanently changes the speech and language characteristics of autism.

2. Some **antipsychotic drugs** (*see* Psychiatric Disorders) may decrease the stereotypic, repetitive utterances.

F. Alternative Treatment

Recently it has been suggested that through typing or pointing some autistic persons may demonstrate they can communicate, but only with a facilitator who supports the wrist or elbow of the autistic person. With this support the autistic individual supposedly is able to type or point to words. Unfortunately, the success of **Facilitative Communication** has not been demonstrated. Whether the method is a reliable, valid measure of the autistic person's written communication skills has not been determined at this time.

G. Recommended Readings

Baron-Cohen, S., & Bolton, P. (1993). *Autism, the facts.* New York: Oxford University Press

Biklen, D. (1992). Typing to talk: Facilitated communication. *American Journal of Speech-Language Pathology, 1*(2), 15–17.

Calculator, S. N. (1992). Perhaps the emperor has clothes after all: A response to Biklen. *American Journal of Speech-Language Pathology, 1*(2), 18–20.

VII. ATTENTION DEFICIT HYPERACTIVITY DISORDER (ADHD) (ADD)

A. Definition/Cause

1. Individuals with Attention Deficit Hyperactivity Disorder (ADHD) demonstrate inappropriate degrees of inattention, impulsivity, and hyperactivity. Many children with ADHD are at risk for speech and language impairment.

2. The cause of ADHD is unknown but a familial component is suspected.

B. General Features, Symptoms, and Signs

1. Inattention, impulsivity, and hyperactivity are observed in all environments—home, school, work, and social situations. Short attention span, restlessness, distractibility, and emotional lability are frequently observed.

2. Symptoms may worsen when sustained attention is required or may be absent when the individual is under strict control: for example, in a one-on-one situation.

3. The child with ADHD may give the impression of not listening, and may often blurt out an answer to a question before the question is completed. In the classroom, the child may begin to work on an assignment before the complete instructions are stated. Fidgeting, twisting, wiggling, squirming, and excessive talking often are observed.

4. ADHD is more prevalent in males than females. In approximately 50% of cases, onset is before 4 years of age. Frequently, the disorder goes unrecognized until a child enters school. School failure is a major complication.

5. ADHD tends to persist into adolescence and adulthood and may negatively influence social relationships, choice of career, and job success and satisfaction. ADHD should be considered a lifetime problem.

Persons with ADHD often fidget with their hands or feet or squirm in their seats. This symptom in adolescents may be limited to subjective feelings of restlessness. The child with ADHD may not remain in a chair when required to do so, is easily distracted by extraneous stimuli, has difficulty awaiting turns in games, and does not follow through on instructions. In addition, these children have difficulty sustaining attention in tasks or play activities and they shift from one uncompleted activity to another. An inability to play quietly, excessive talking and interrupting, and losing things necessary for tasks or activities have been noted. The child or adult with ADHD often engages in physically dangerous activities without considering the possible consequences.

C. General Features, Symptoms, and Signs of Communication Impairment

A variety of behaviors affecting communication have been reported, including delayed language development, disordered articulation, and impaired cognition.

D. Pharmacologic Treatment

1. **Stimulants (Psychostimulants, Central Nervous System [CNS] Stimulants)** are the most effective and least toxic of the medicines used to treat ADHD.

    a. Amphetamine-like drugs reduce symptoms in 80% of affected children.

    b. Whether or not stimulants improve cognitive function and increase overall academic achievement remains controversial.

    c. **Dextroamphetamine (D-Amphetamine, Dexedrine®)** Initially, dextroamphetamine was the only effective agent available. It is still prescribed for some individuals.
       (1) **Desired effects of D-amphetamine** are sustained attention and decreased impulsivity and hyperactivity.
       (2) **Undesirable effects: Anorexia** (loss of appetite), **weight loss, sleep disturbance** (insomnia). A potential for **abuse compared with other stimulants available, headache,**

abdominal pain, depressed mood, heightened anxiety, and **lack of spontaneity** are milder side effects of dextroamphetamine. More severe side effects are **hypertension, cerebral hemorrhage, arrhythmia, convulsions, coma, confusion, fever** and **tremor**. In addition, **bizarre behavior, hallucinations, paranoia, agitation, anxiety,** and **symptoms of mania** and **depression** are psychiatric symptoms caused by amphetamines.

2. **Methylphenidate (Ritalin®).** The primary action that calms hyperactivity is not known. Ritalin® may increase the release of the neurotransmitter norepinepherine. Often, Ritalin® is the drug of choice for ADHD, probably because it has less potential for abuse than dextroamphetamine.

   a. **Desired effects** of Ritalin® are **improved alertness and concentration** and **increased attention span.**

   b. **Undesirable effects** are **anorexia, insomnia,** and **nervousness. Growth retardation** may occur with prolonged use, but methylphenidate does not adversely affect ultimate height. (*See* Table 5–7 for a complete list of adverse effects of methylphenidate.)

Table 5–7. Side effects of methylphenidate (Ritalin®).

Nervousness

Insomnia

Anorexia, weight loss

Growth retardation

Dizziness

Dyskinesia

Skin rash

Gastrointestinal disturbance

Hypertension

Palpitation and changes in heart and pulse rate

Headache

Seizures

c. **General remarks**. The ideal dosage depends on the age of the patient and the patient's reaction to the drug. Ritalin is prescribed with extreme caution for patients with seizure disorder because of its propensity for causing seizures. The safety and effectiveness of the drug have not been established for children under the age of 6 years. Persons more than age 60 years may be susceptible to developing **nervousness, agitation, insomnia, hypertension, angina,** or **disturbance of heart rhythm** as a result of taking Ritalin.

3. **Pemoline (Cylert®)** has the lowest abuse potential of all stimulants.

   a. **Desired effects** are similar to those of methylphenidate and include **improved alertness and concentration**, and **increased attention span**.

   b. **Undesirable effects. Insomnia** and **anorexia** are common. Less frequent side effects are **dizziness, drowsiness, headache, depression, hallucinations, skin rash,** and **nausea and other gastrointestinal distress**. After several months of treatment, liver function may be affected. This may reverse if the drug is withdrawn. **Psychotic behavior** may be observed if pemoline is not used appropriately.

4. **Tricyclic Antidepressants**. Although stimulants are the drugs of choice for treatment of ADHD, antidepressants sometimes are prescribed for older children or for adults who experience associated anxiety or mood disorders (*see* Depression). For **desired** and **undesirable effects** of antidepressant drugs, *see* Depression.

5. **Benzodiazepines** may be prescribed for persons with ADHD. *See* Anxiety Disorders for **desired** and **undesirable effects** of benzodiazapines.

E. Effects of the Drugs on Communication

1. When effective, stimulants improve concentration and attention. Performance on cognition and memory tasks improves with stimulant drugs.
2. **Vocal tremor** and **rapid speech rate** are reported side effects of dextroamphetamine.
3. **Phonic tics** have been noted as a side effect of pemoline.

F. Alternative Treatments

> Although prescription drugs may improve the attention of children and adults with ADHD, it is generally agreed that the drugs alone do not help children learn.

1. **Individual and family counseling** and/or **psychotherapy focusing on enhancing school performance** and **encouraging behavior suitable for the classroom** often are advantageous. The child with ADHD may need professional counseling in young adulthood and beyond.

2. **Concise**, rather than extended, **reprimands** for misbehaving and **positive reinforcement** for desirable behavior have been the most effective facilitators for learning for children with ADHD. Teachers and parents are encouraged to use these techniques as an adjunct to drug therapy.

3. **Neurofeedback**, a specialized form of **biofeedback**, may have applications for ADHD. Training the individual with ADHD to reduce the alpha waves associated with quiet states, while sustaining the theta waves associated with active states, has resulted in a reduction in anxiety reactions and a return to normal waveforms and sustained attention.

4. **Cognitive therapy emphasizing tasks designed to improve attention** is effective in some cases.

5. **Speech-language therapy** can be beneficial.

G. Recommended Readings

Baron-Cohen, S. & Bolton, P. (1993). *Autism: the Facts*. New York: Oxford University Press.

Biederman, J., Faraone, S. V., Spencer, T., Wilens, T., Norman, D., Lapey, K. A., Mick, E., Lehman, B. K., & Doyle, A. (1993). Patterns of psychiatric comorbidity, cognition and psychosocial functioning in adults with attention deficit hyperactivity disorder. *American Journal of Psychiatry, 150*(19), 1792–1797.

Diagnostic and statistical manual of mental disorders (DSM IV-R). (1994). (4th ed: revised). Washington, DC: American Psychiatric Association.

Green, G. H. (1993, November). Eyes rolled back in his head, he contemplates the mind/body problem. Life without stress. *Gazette-Journal*, Reno, Nevada, 6.

Kennedy, P., Terdal, L., & Fusetti, L. (1993). *The hyperactive child book*. New York: St. Martin's Press.

Olson, J. (1991). *Clinical pharmacology made ridiculously simple*. Miami, FL. Medmaster, Inc.

Ward, M. F., Wender, P., & Reimherr, F. W. (1993). The Wender Utah Rating Scale: An aid in the retrospective diagnosis of childhood ADHD. American *Journal of Psychiatry, 150*, 885–890.

CHAPTER

6

Idiopathic Speech and Voice Specific Disorders

This chapter covers two idiopathic communication disorders. For each, we provide a definition, discuss the general features, symptoms, and signs; describe the features, symptoms, and signs of communication impairment; list pharmacologic treatments; and discuss the influence drug treatment may have on communication.

I. STUTTERING

A Definition/Cause

   1. Stuttering has been defined as the involuntary repetition and prolongation of speech sounds and syllables that the individual struggles to end.

2. **Developmental stuttering** begins in childhood or early adolescence. Prevalence is about 1% in the adult population.

3. **Neurogenic dysfluency** has a sudden onset and almost always is associated with gross impairment of brain function resulting from traumatic brain injury, stroke, brain tumor, or other insult to the brain.

4. **Psychogenic dysfluency** is neither developmentally nor neurologically based. It occurs in adulthood, is of sudden onset, and is temporally linked to some form of psychological trauma or cumulative psychological stress.

5. Theories regarding the etiology of stuttering have ranged from "dryness of the tongue and faulty anatomy of the oral cavity" to "expression of unconscious conflicts and impaired learning." Possibly a developmental disorder of the central nervous system is the cause. Still another theory is that stuttering is a subtle abnormality of central auditory functioning or sensory-motor processing.

B. General Features, Symptoms, and Signs

In addition to the primary symptoms, (*see* Features, Symptoms, and Signs of Communication Impairment), there may be tremors of the lips and jaw, rapid blinking, jerking movements of the head, arm, or upper trunk, and other manifestations of the person's struggle to speak.

C. Features, Symptoms, and Signs of Communication Impairment

Frequent repetitions or prolongations of sounds or syllables that markedly impair the fluency of speech are signs of stuttering.

D. Pharmacologic Treatment

A wide range of pharmacologic agents has been tried. Table 6–1 provides a list of authors who have reported cases or results of controlled studies of drugs used to attempt to control stuttering. Also included in Table 6–1 are the drugs used, a brief description of subjects studied, and the results or conclusions reported.

E. Effects of Drugs on Communication

To date, no agent has emerged as the drug of choice for control of stuttering, and the search for effective drug therapy for stuttering continues.

Table 6–1. Reports of drugs used to control stuttering.

Investigators	Drug(s)	Subjects	Results
Kent (1963)	Tranquilizers: reserpine chlorpromazine meprobamate atarax	"Many adults"	No significant reduction with or without speech therapy
Wells & Malcolm (1971)	haloperidol antihistamines	36 adults	12 subjects who completed the 8-week trial maintained improvement on one of three measures of stuttering severity
Quinn & Peachy (1973)	haloperidol antihistamines	18 adults	Improvement in 4 subjects
Murray, Kelly, Campbell, & Stefanik (1977)	haloperidol	26 adults	Significant improvement
Brady, Burns, & Kuruvilla (1978)	haloperidol	12 adults	Improvement in 9 subjects
Prins, Mandelkorn, & Cerf	haloperidol	14 subjects, aged 7–14 years	Significantly reduced dysfluencies and increased speaking rate
Zachariah (1980)	verapamil, a calcium channel blocker	50 adults	Good response in 42 subjects
McLean & McLean (1985)	phenytoin	1 head injured adult	Patient began to stutter as a result of taking the drug
Goldstein & Goldberg (1986)	phenelzine	1 adult female	Induced speech blockage

(continued)

Table 6–1. *(continued)*

Investigators	Drug(s)	Subjects	Results
Goldstein (1987)	carbamazepine	1 adult male with a moderate stutter, 1 adult female with a very severe stutter	Striking improvement
Hays (1987)	bethanecol chloride	2 adults	Improvement
Adler & Leong (1987)	propranolol (beta blocker)	2 adult males aged 43 and 69 years	Resolution of symptoms
Brumfitt & Peake (1988)	verapamil	14 adults aged 19–47 years	No evidence of improvement
Rosenfield (1988)	carbamazepine	3 adult stutters	No response
Brady, Price, McAllister, & Dietrich (1989)	verapamil	10 adults aged 30–70 years	Improvement in 9 subjects
Burris, Riggs, & Brinkley (1990)	betaxlol (beta blocker)	1 male, aged 50 years	Striking improvement
Costa (1992)	mianserine, an antidepressant	19 subjects	11 subjects responded well (They stuttered less.) Six subjects reported a side effect of drowsiness
Harvey, Culatta, Halikas, Sorenson, Luxenberg, & Pearson (1992)	carbamazepine	12 adults who received 800 mg; 8 adults who received 400 mg.	No change in percentage of words stuttered, no reading improvement or improvement in spontaneous speech rate. Subjective reports of decreased struggle characteristics. Improvement as measured by ratings of naive judges.

(continued)

Table 6–1. *(continued)*

Investigators	Drug(s)	Subjects	Results
Kampman & Brady (1993)	bethanechol	Adult stutterers	Drug not superior to placebo; however, 2 patients who responded favorably continued with the medication and remained more fluent after taking the drug for 6 months.
Oberlander, Schneier, & Liebowitz (1993)	phenelzine (MAO inhibitor)	1 male, aged 24 years	After 6 weeks on the drug, the patient ingested vodka for 10 days and became manic with rapid and pressured speech. In his manic state, he no longer stuttered.

F. Alternative Treatments

A variety of treatments for stuttering have been reported. Among them are:

1. Chemical or surgical means of controlling the "dryness of the tongue." Hippocrates believed tongue dryness was the cause of stuttering.

2. Cauteries and blisters were applied to the neck and behind the ears in sixteenth-century Italy.

3. Surgery on the tongue, frenulum, or uvula was a popular procedure in the nineteenth century.

4. Psychosocial and behavioral treatments, among them operant conditioning and psychoanalytic psychotherapy.

5. A wide variety of speech therapy techniques have been used with varying degrees of success.

G. Recommended Readings

Boone, D. R., & Plante, E. (1993). *Human communication and its disorders* (2nd ed.), Englewood Cliffs, NJ: Prentice Hall.

Brady, J. P. (1991). The pharmacology of stuttering: A critical review. *American Journal of Psychiatry, 148,* 1309–1316.

Deal, J. L., & Cannito, M. P. (1991). Acquired neurogenic dysfluency. In D. Vogel & M. P. Cannito, (Eds.), *Treating disordered speech motor control: For clinicians by clinicians* (Vol. 6, pp. 217–239). Austin, TX: Pro-Ed.

Deal, J. L., & Doro, J. M. (1987). Episodic hysterical stuttering. *Journal of Speech and Hearing Disorders, 52,* 229–300.

Rosenfield, D. B. (1991). Pharmacologic approaches to speech motor disorders. In D. Vogel & M. P. Cannito, (Eds.) *Treating disordered speech motor control: For clinicians by clinicians* (Vol. 6, pp. 111–152). Austin, TX: Pro-Ed.

II. SPASMODIC DYSPHONIA

A. Definition/Cause

1 Spasmodic dysphonia (SD) has been described as a devastating neurologic voice disorder of unknown etiology with a variable clinical presentation and a variable response to treatment. Some theories evoke psychiatric and organic etiologies, including conversion reaction—the person with SD is choking off attempts to communicate—essential tremor of laryngeal muscles accompanied by voice arrest, and demyelination of the recurrent laryngeal nerve.

2. SD appears to affect men and women in approximately equal proportions.

3. Onset has been reported as early as adolescence, but the average age of onset is approximately 50 years of age.

B. General Features, Symptoms, and Signs

Slow, insidious onset is common, although some patients with SD report a sudden onset traced to an important event in their lives.

C. Features, Symptoms, and Signs of Communication Impairment

1. Voice characteristics are staccato, jerky, squeezed, effortful, strained-strangled, or groaning vocalizations. Some behaviors, such as laughing, crying, moaning, coughing, and singing, may be

normal as are periods of voice free of symptoms of SD. Some patients can prolong vowels at high pitch levels with no evidence of vocal pathology.

2. **Adductor spasmodic dysphonia** is characterized by forceful, involuntary approximation of the vocal folds. This interrupts the airstream and produces the strained, harsh, choppy voice that is often described. **Abductor spasmodic dysphonia,** another type of SD, is characterized by forceful, involuntary separation of the vocal folds, causing breathy interruptions in speech.

D. Pharmacologic Treatment

1. **Botulinum toxin (Botox®)** is a complex protein produced by the anaerobic bacterium, *Clostridium botulinum.* The toxin causes paralysis by blocking the presynaptic release of acetylcholine at the neuromuscular junction. Although well known as a cause of serious and often fatal paralysis acquired through ingestion of contaminated food, it has been found that the blocking effect alleviates muscle spasm or weakens a muscle for therapeutic purposes. Injections of botulinum toxin have provided substantial relief of symptoms of SD that has lasted for weeks to months.

   a. **Desirable effect** of botulinum toxin is **relief from the symptoms.**

   b. **Undesirable effects.** Persistent complications of botulinum toxin injections are rare, and serious side effects are uncommon. Influenza-like syndrome has been reported, but is rare. Some patients have developed antibodies to the toxin. Relief from symptoms of SD is transient, and repeated injections are required.

2. **Methazolamine (Neptazane®)** is a drug used typically to dry the aqueous humor of the eye. For reasons not clear at this time, the drug been shown to affect the symptoms of adductor spasmodic dysphonia. More evidence of beneficial effects is needed before methazolamine is considered a drug of choice for the treatment of SD.

E. Effects of the Drugs on Communication

1. Botulinum toxin therapy is effective for relieving symptoms and restoring fluency in cases of adductor spasmodic dysphonia, but it is less effective in all but a few carefully selected cases of abductor spasmodic dysphonia. In abductor spasmodic dysphonia, there is risk of bilateral abductor paralysis with airway obstruction if the posterior cricoarytenoid muscles are injected.

2. The effects of botulinum toxin are not permanent. Symptoms return, and the patient must undergo frequent injections.

3. The long-term effects of methazolamine on communication are unknown at this time.

F. Alternative Treatments

1. **Surgical procedures.** Resecting or crushing the recurrent laryngeal nerve has provided a permanent, but more often, a temporary solution to the problem of adductor spasmodic dysphonia.

2. **Voice therapy.** Although SD has been reported to be resistant to voice therapy, some patients have considered compensatory strategies learned in speech therapy sessions to be beneficial.

G. Recommended Readings

Cannito, M. P. (1991). Neurobiological interpretations of spasmodic dysphonia. In D. Vogel & M. P. Cannito, (Eds.) *Treating disordered speech motor control: For clinicians by clinicians* (Vol. 6, pp. 275–317). Austin, TX. Pro-Ed.

Dedo, H. H., & Izdebski, K. (1983). Problems with surgical (RLN section) treatment of spastic dysphonia. *Largyngoscope, 93,* 268–271.

Hartman, D. E., Abbs, J. M., Vishwanat, A. K., Bouri, J. V., Beardsley, C. W., & Rooney, B. (1994, March). *Response of essential voice tremor and spasmodic dysphonia to methazolamide (Neptazane®).* Paper presented at Sedona, Arizona, Conference on Motor Speech.

National Institutes of Health Consensus Development Conference Statement, (1990). Clinical use of Botulinum toxin. *Archives of Neurology, 48,* 1294–1298.

GLOSSARY

Terms Related to Medical Conditions and Management

Acetylcholine. The neurotransmitter released at the synapses of parasympathetic nerves and at neuromuscular junctions. After relaying a nerve impulse, acetylcholine is rapidly broken down by the enzyme, cholinesterase.

Agranulocytosis. A disorder in which there is a severe acute deficiency of certain blood cells (neutrophils) as a result of damage to the bone marrow by toxic drugs or chemicals. It is characterized by fever, with ulceration of the mouth and throat, and may rapidly lead to prostration and death. Agranulocytosis can be a side effect of certain psychotropic drugs.

Akinesia. A loss of normal muscle tone or responsiveness.

Akathisia. Restless overactivity, involuntary movements induced by antipsychotic drugs.

Allergic Reaction; Allergy. An undesirable response occurring in individuals producing antibodies that react with drugs. Allergic reactions may appear as skin rash, fever, painful joints, breathing difficulty, and collapse of circulation. Drug allergies can develop gradually, or can appear suddenly. Some allergic reactions are life-threatening.

Amenorrhea. Absence or stopping of the menstrual periods. Amenorrhea is a side effect of certain drugs and is a symptom of depression.

Amyotrophy. A progressive loss of muscle bulk associated with weakness of these muscles. It is a feature of chronic neuropathy. Amyotrophy combined with spasticity characterizes motor neuron disease.

Anaphylaxis. An abnormal reaction to a particular antigen in which histamine is released from the tissues and causes either local or widespread symptoms. An allergic attack is an example of localized anaphylaxis. Rarer, but much more serious, is anaphylactic shock in which widespread histamine release causes swelling, constrictions of the bronchioles, heart failure, circulatory collapse and, sometimes, death.

Aneurysm. A balloon-like swelling in the wall of an artery. Aneurysms within the brain can be congenital, and if they burst, they may cause a subarachnoid hemorrhage.

Antibodies. Blood proteins that combine with substances that are foreign to the body. Antibodies either can be protective or injurious. Protective antibodies destroy bacteria and neutralize toxins, while injurious antibodies, combined with foreign substances, cause allergic reactions.

Anticholinergics, anticholinergic drugs. Drugs that inhibit the action of acetylcholine. Side effects of anticholinergics include dry mouth, blurred vision, and dizziness. More serious side effects are impaired cognition, constipation, urinary retention, and precipitation of untreated glaucoma.

Anticholinesterase. A substance that inhibits the action of cholinesterase, the enzyme responsible for the breakdown of the neurotransmitter, acetylcholine. Anticholinesterase allows acetylcholine to continue transmitting nerve impulses.

Anticonvulsant. A drug that prevents or reduces the severity of seizures in various types of epilepsy. The choice of anticonvulsant is dictated by the type of seizure and the response to the drug. Some anticonvulsants are used for all types of seizures, others are type-specific.

Antidepressant. A drug that alleviates the symptoms of depression. The most widely prescribed are the tricyclic antidepressants. Another main group of antidepressants are the MAO inhibitors; these have more severe side effects than the tricyclics. New classes of antidepressants are discussed in the text.

Aplastic anemia. A disorder of white blood cell production.

Arrhythmia. A deviation from the normal rhythm (sinus rhythm) of the heart. Arrhythmias may be intermittent or continuous, and may arise from various causes including the adverse effect of certain drugs.

Arthralgia. Pain in a joint without swelling or arthritis.

Asthenia. Weakness or loss of strength.

Astrocytoma. A brain tumor in which all grades of malignancy occur— from slow growing, with nearly normal cells, to rapidly growing, highly invasive tumors.

Ataxia. Unsteady gait with incoordination of movement. Ataxic (cere- bellar) dysarthria may co-exist with the unsteady gait.

Atrophy. The wasting away of a normally developed organ or tissue due to degeneration of cells.

Autism. A severe psychiatric disorder of childhood manifested by severe difficulties in communicating, forming relationships, developing language, and using abstract concepts.

Autoimmune Disease. A disease thought to be caused by inflammation and destruction of tissues by the body's own antibodies.

Barbiturate. Drugs derived from barbituric acid that depress the activity of the CNS. Slow acting barbiturates may be used to control seizures.

Benign. Description of a tumor that does not invade or destroy the tis- sue in which it originates. Benign tumors do not metastasize. Often the term "benign" is used to describe a tumor that is not cancerous.

Beta blocker. A drug that prevents stimulation of receptors of the nerves of the sympathetic nervous system, and therefore decreases the activity of the heart. Beta blockers may be used to control abnormal heart rhythms, to treat angina, and to reduce high blood pressure.

Blood-brain barrier. The mechanism whereby the circulating blood is kept separate from the tissue fluids surrounding the brain cells.

Blood dyscrasia. An abnormal state of the blood, usually due to abnor- mal development or metabolism.

Bone marrow depression. Bone marrow is the tissue contained within the internal cavities of the bones. At birth, these cavities are filled with blood-forming tissue, but in later life the marrow in the limb bones is replaced by fat. Depression of bone marrow is a side effect of certain drugs.

Bradykinesia. A symptom of parkinsonism manifested by difficulty in initiating movements, slowness in executing movements, and an inability to make adjustments to posturing of the body.

Brand name. The registered trade name given to a drug by its manufacturer. The brand name designates that the drug is protected by a patent or copyright.

Bruise, contusion. An area of skin discoloration caused by the escape of blood from ruptured underlying vessels following injury. The drawing off of blood through a needle may be necessary to aid the healing of very severe bruises.

Bureau of Drugs. A division of the United States Food and Drug Administration responsible for the regulation of drugs available to patients. The efficacy of new drugs must be proven before the drugs can be prescribed by physicians.

Cause-effect relationship. A possible association between a drug and a side effect. Often it is not possible to establish that a drug is responsible for an effect. Cause-effect relationships are more likely to be established when the effect immediately follows the administration of the drug and when the adverse effect disappears after the drug is discontinued and reappears after subsequent use. In establishing cause-effect relationships, consideration must be given to progression of disease, the interval between the administration and a reaction to the drug, and the interaction between drugs if more than one is taken.

Chemotherapy. The prevention or treatment of a disease by the use of chemical substances. The term is restricted to drugs used to control cancer.

Clonic. Relating to or resembling clonus. The term is used to describe the rhythmic limb movements in epilepsy.

Compliance. The taking of medication as the prescriber intended. Conversely, *noncompliance* is either, consciously or through error or though misunderstanding, *not* taking the medication as intended by the prescriber.

Contraindication. Any factor that makes it unwise to pursue a particular treatment. For example, a specific condition may be a contraindication against the use of a certain drug.

Craniotomy. Surgical removal of a portion of the skull to expose the cortex and meninges for inspection or biopsy. Craniotomy is performed to relieve excessive intracranial pressure, as in subdural hematoma.

Cushing's syndrome. A condition resulting from excess amounts of corticosteroid hormones in the body. Symptoms include weight gain, reddening of the face and neck, excess growth of body and facial hair, raised blood pressure, loss of mineral from bone (osteoporosis), raised blood glucose levels, and, sometimes, cognitive disturbances.

Demyelination. A process that selectively damages the myelin sheath in the nervous system. Affecting the nerve fibers supported by the myelin, demyelination may be the primary disorder, as in multiple sclerosis, or may occur secondary to brain injury or stroke.

Diaphoresis. The process of sweating, especially excessive sweating.

Diplopia. Double vision. The simultaneous awareness of two images of one object. Usually diplopia is due to a disturbance in the coordination of muscles that move the eye. Covering one eye will stop the diplopia.

Disease. A disorder with a specific cause and recognizable signs and symptoms. A bodily abnormality or failure to function normally, except when resulting directly from physical injury.

Disorientation. A state produced by loss of awareness of space, time, or person. Disorientation can be a consequence of drugs, anxiety, or organic disease.

Dispensary. A place where medicines are made up by a pharmacist and dispensed to patients.

Drug. A medicine used in medical practice. A chemical entity that provokes a specific response when it is placed in a biological system.

Drug class. A group of drugs similar in chemistry, method of action, and use. Drugs within the same class can produce similar beneficial effects and side effects. Significant variations may occur that allow the physician to choose a particular drug if certain beneficial actions are desired or certain side effects are to be minimized or avoided.

Gait. The manner in which a person walks. In neurological disease, the gait is often unsteady or uncoordinated. A staggering gait indicates alcohol or barbiturate intoxication or can be an indication of cerebellar disease.

Gamma-aminobutyic acid (GABA). An amino acid in the brain, where it acts as an inhibitory neurotransmitter.

Generic name. The official, common, or public name used to designate a specific drug by its principal active ingredients. Many drugs have no brand name. Generics, as a rule, are less expensive than brand name drugs and may be, but not always are, identical to a prescribed brand name drug.

Glioblastoma multiforme. An aggressive type of brain tumor. Its rapid enlargement destroys normal brain cells, with a progressive loss of function. The resultant raised intracranial pressure causes headache, vomiting, and drowsiness.

Glioma. A term frequently used for all tumors that arise in the central nervous system, including astrocytomas, oligodendrogliomas, and medulloblastomas. Tumors of low-grade malignancy produce symptoms by their pressure on surrounding structures. Those of high-grade malignancy may be invasive.

Granulocytopenia. A reduction of the number of granulocytes (a type of white cell) in the blood.

Hallucination. A false perception of something that is not really there. Hallucinations may be visual, auditory, tactile, or of taste or smell. They may be provoked by psychological illness, for example, schizophrenia, or by physical disorders involving the brain, for example, temporal lobe epilepsy or stroke; or they may be caused by drugs or sensory deprivation.

Hemorrhagic pancreatitis. Pancreatitis is an inflammation of the pancreas, a compound gland that lies beneath the stomach. In hemorrhagic pancreatitis, there is bleeding into the pancreas. Possible causes are gall stones or alcoholism.

Hepatitis. An inflammation of the liver caused by viruses, toxic substances, or immunological abnormalities.

Hepatotoxicity, hepatotoxic reaction. Damage or destruction to liver cells. Certain drugs can cause hepatotoxicity.

Hirsutism. The presence of coarse hair on the face, chest, upper back, or abdomen as a side effect of certain drugs.

Hypersensitivity. Overresponsiveness to drug action. Intolerance to even small doses. Some individuals who are allergic to a particular drug will be allergic to other drugs that are closely related in chemical composition (*see* **Drug Class**).

Hypoxic-ischemic insult. A deficiency of oxygen in the tissues, leading to ischemic insult.

Hypnotic. A drug used primarily to induce sleep. Antihistamines, barbiturates, and benzodiazepines are classes of drugs that produce hypnotic effects.

Hypothermia. Accidental reduction of body temperature below the normal range in the absence of reflex actions, for example, shivering. Hypothermia occurs most often in infants and the elderly. It can be a side effect of certain drugs.

Iatrogenic. Description of a condition resulting from treatment, as either an unforeseen or inevitable side effect.

Idiopathic. A disease or condition the cause of which is unknown. Idiopathic diseases or conditions may arise spontaneously.

Immunosuppressant drug. A drug that reduces the body's resistance to infection and other foreign bodies by suppressing the immune system. Because immunity is lowered during treatment with immunosuppressants there is an increased risk of infection. Immunosuppressant drugs are used for treating chronic autoimmune diseases.

Injection. Introduction into the body of drugs or other fluids by means of a syringe. Usually these drugs, if taken orally, would be destroyed by the digestive process. Common routes for injection are intracutaneous (into the skin), subcutaneous (below the skin), intramuscular (into a muscle for slow absorption), and intravenous (into a vein for rapid absorption).

Insomnia. Inability to fall asleep or to remain asleep for an adequate length of time to eliminate tiredness. Insomnia may be associated with disease or may occur as a side effect of certain drugs.

Interaction. An unwanted change in the response to a drug that results when another drug is administered at the same time. Drug interactions can enhance the effect of either drug, reduce drug effectiveness, or produce a toxic response. (*see* **Toxicity**).

Intervention study. A comparison of the outcome between two or more groups of patients that are deliberately subjected to different drug regimens. Patients in the control group have no active treatment. Patients in the experimental groups are subjected to active drug treatment. In a randomized controlled trial, all subjects are assigned randomly to control or experimental groups. Ideally, the study should be a double blind cross-over design in which neither the patient nor the experimenter assessing the outcome is aware of the group to which the patient has been assigned. In these studies in which two drugs or a drug and a placebo are administered, study patients exchange treatments after a prearranged period.

Jaundice. A yellow coloration of the skin and the white of the eyes that occurs when excessive bile pigments accumulate in the blood as a result of impaired liver function. Jaundice may be a sign of disease or a reaction to a particular drug.

Kayser-Fleischer ring. A brownish-yellow ring in the outer rim of the cornea of the eye caused by a deposit of copper granules. This sign is diagnostic of Wilson's disease. When well developed these rings may be seen by the naked eye, but if faint, they may detected only by specialized ophthalmological examination.

Leukopenia. A reduction of the number of white blood cells (leukocytes) in the blood.

MAO Inhibitor. A drug that prevents the activity of the enzyme monoamine oxidase (MAO) in brain tissue and therefore affects mood. Their use may be restricted because of the severity of their side effects.

Medication. A substance administered by mouth, applied to the skin, or introduced into the body for the purpose of treatment.

Meningioma. A tumor arising from the meninges, the fibrous coverings of the brain and spinal cord.

Mitral valve prolapse. The mitral valve is located in the heart and consists of two flaps attached to the walls at the opening between the left atrium and the left ventricle. It allows the blood to pass through the atrium to the ventricle but prevents backward flow. Mitral valve prolapse refers to a downward displacement of the valve from its normal position, and, usually is the result of weakening of its supporting tissues.

Mydriasis. A widening of the pupil that occurs normally in dim light. The most common causes of prolonged mydriasis are drug therapy or injuries to the eye.

Neoplasm (of the brain). An abnormal multiplication of brain cells. This forms edema that compresses or destroys healthy brain cells and, because the skill is rigid, increases pressure on the brain.

Nephrotic syndrome. A condition in which, due to edema, there is great loss of protein in the urine, reduced levels of albumin in the blood, and generalized swelling of the tissues.

Nephritis. Inflammation of the kidney. Also referred to as Bright's disease.

Neuroblastoma. A malignant tumor composed of embryonic nerve cells.

Neurofibromatosis. A congenital disease typified by numerous benign tumors growing from the fibrous coverings of nerves. Tumors may occur in the spinal canal, where they may press on the spinal cord. Pigmented patches on the skin are found in a large number of cases. This condition is also known as von Recklinghausen's disease.

Neuroleptic malignant syndrome. A rare, serious, potentially fatal reaction to antipsychotic drugs.

Neurotransmitter. A chemical substance released from nerve endings to transmit impulses across synapses to other muscles, nerves, or glands.

Optic neuropathy. Neuropathy is any disease of the peripheral nerves, usually causing weakness and numbness. Optic neuropathy refers to disease of the optic nerve and, often, is diagnostic of multiple sclerosis.

Orphan drug. A drug used for treating relatively rare conditions and thus has no potential for making a profit for the drug manufacturer. Many requirements of the FDA are omitted. There are more than 100 orphan drugs.

Orthostatic hypotension (Postural hypotension). Low blood pressure related to body position or posture. The blood pressure may be normal when lying down, but upon sitting or standing sudden sensations of dizziness, lightheadedness, and feeling faint are experienced, resulting in the quick return to the lying down position. The condition is due to inadequate oxygen supply and, therefore, inadequate blood flow to the brain. This results in an abnormal delay in the rise of blood pressure that occurs as the body adjusts the circulation to the upright position.

Over-the-counter drugs (OTCs) (Non-prescription drugs). Drugs that may be purchased without prescription. These products should be regarded as medicines that can interact with prescription or other OTC drugs.

Overdose. More than the optimal dosage resulting from a variety of sources. Overdose can result from the accumulation of prescribed daily doses of a drug or can occur with accidental ingestion of drugs, for example, by children or by adults with suicidal intention.

Palilalia. A disorder in which a word is rapidly and involuntarily repeated. It occurs in Gilles de la Tourette syndrome and other disorders of the extrapyramidal system.

Palliative. A medicine or procedure that gives temporary relief from symptoms but does not cure the underlying disease.

Pallidectomy. A neurosurgical procedure designed to destroy or modify the effects of the globus pallidus. This procedure is used for relief of parkinsonism and other conditions in which involuntary movements are prominent.

Paradoxical reaction. An unexpected drug response that is inconsistent with known pharmacology. These reactions may be due to individual sensitivity, and appear to be more common in children and the elderly.

Paraparesis. Weakness of both legs, resulting from disease of the nervous system.

Parenteral. Administration of a drug through other than oral administration; for example, by injection.

Pedal edema. Swelling of the foot.

Pharmacodynamics. The interaction of drugs with cells.

Pharmacokinetics. The processes of absorption, distribution, metabolism, and excretion of a drug.

Pharmacology. The science of development and use of medicines, including the composition of medicines and their actions in animals and man.

Pharmacy. The preparation and dispensing of drugs. A place registered to dispense medicines.

Phenylketonuria. A congenital defect of protein metabolism that causes excessive amounts of the amino acid phenylalanine in the blood. The condition causes damage to the nervous system, and leads to severe mental retardation. The responsible gene is recessive so that a child is affected only if both parents are carriers of the defective gene.

Photophobia. An abnormal intolerance of light, in which exposure to light causes intense discomfort to the eyes. Tight contraction of the eyelids and other reactions may be used to avoid the light. Photophobia may be associated with dilation of the pupils as a reaction to certain drugs.

Placebo. A drug that is ineffective but may relieve symptoms because the patient believes it will. New drugs are tested against placebos in clinical trials. The placebo response is one that occurs even in the absence of any pharmacologically active substance.

Plasmapheresis. The method of removing a quantity of plasma from a patient's blood. After the plasma is removed, the blood cells are transfused back into the patient.

Polypharmacy. Treatment with more than one type of medicine.

Prescription. A written direction from a medical practitioner to a pharmacist for preparing and dispensing a drug.

Prognosis. Assessment of the future course and outcome of a patient's condition, based on knowledge of the outcome of the condition in other patients. The patient's general health, age, and sex are considered in the prognosis.

Psychosis. A severe psychiatric illness in which the patient loses contact with reality.

Ptosis. The drooping of the upper eyelid, for which there are several causes, including a disorder of the occulomotor nerve or a widespread fatigable weakness.

Radiotherapy. The treatment of a disease with penetrating radiation which may be produced by machines or radioactive isotopes. Beams of radiation may be directed at a diseased organ from a distance; or radioactive material in the form of needles, wires, or pellets, may be implanted in the body. Many forms of cancer are destroyed by radiation; however, radiation can damage normal tissues.

Resting tremor. A rhythmic to and fro movement of the extremity.

Rigidity. Increased resistance to passive movements of a limb that is present throughout the range of movement.

Sepsis. Destruction of tissues by disease-causing bacteria or their toxins.

Side effect. An undesirable response to a drug. The majority of side effects are minor annoyances and inconveniences; but some are counterproductive in disease management, and some are potentially dangerous.

Sign. An indication of a disease or a disorder noticed by someone other than the patient, often by the physician.

Spasm. A sustained muscle contraction.

Spasticity. Resistance to the passive movement of a limb that is maximal at the beginning of the movement, giving way as more pressure is applied. Spasticity is a symptom of damage to the corticospinal tracts in the brain or spinal cord, and usually is accompanied by weakness in the affected limb.

Stereotaxic technique. A surgical procedure in which a deep-seated area in the brain is operated on after its position has been established accurately by three-dimensional measurements. The operation may be performed using an electrical current or by heat, cold, or mechanical techniques.

Stupor. A condition of near unconsciousness with no apparent mental activity and reduced ability to respond to stimulation.

Subarachnoid hemorrhage. Bleeding into the subarachnoid space surrounding the brain which causes severe headache with stiffness of the neck. The usual source is a cerebral aneurysm.

Symptom. An indication of a disease or disorder noticed by the patient, her- or himself.

Symptomatology. Collectively, the symptoms of a disease.

Syncope. Fainting, that is, loss of consciousness induced by a temporarily insufficient flow of blood to brain. Syncope may be caused by an emotional shock, by standing for prolonged periods, by injury with profuse bleeding, or it may be a side effect of a drug. An attack comes on gradually with lightheadedness, sweating, and blurred vision. Typically, recovery is prompt, without any persisting ill effects from the syncope itself.

Tablet. A small disk containing one or more drugs. Tablets are made by compressing a powdered form of the drugs and are taken orally.

Tachycardia. An increase in heart rate to above normal. Tachycardia may be produced by arrythmias.

Tardive dyskinesia. A drug-induced disorder of the nervous system occurring after long-term treatment with psychotropic drugs.

Thalamotomy. Surgery in which a lesion is made in a precise area of the thalamus. Thalamotomy has been used to control psychiatric symptoms of severe anxiety (psychosurgery), in which case, the lesion is made in the dorsomedial nucleus of the thalamus that connects with the frontal lobe. Thalamotomy has been used to control symptoms of Parkinson's disease.

Thrombocytopenia. A reduction in the number of platelets in the blood that may result from failure of platelet production or excessive destruction of platelets. Thrombocytopenia may result in bleeding into the skin, spontaneous bruising, and prolonged bleeding after injury.

Thrombophlebitis. Inflammation of the wall of a vein that may lead to secondary thrombosis occurring within the affected segment of the vein.

Thymoma. A benign or malignant tumor of the thymus gland.

Thyrotropin-releasing hormone (TRH). A hormone-like substance from the hypothalamus that acts on the anterior pituitary gland to stimulate the release of thyroid-stimulating hormone.

Tic. A repeated involuntary movement.

Tolerance. Reduced responsiveness to a drug. Certain medicines or dosages are not effective. A change in the drug or dosage becomes necessary. Side effects may occur, then disappear, during continuous use of a drug.

Toxicity. Having a poisonous effect; potentially lethal. A toxic drug has the potential for dangerously impairing body functions or damaging body tissues. Usually, the larger the dose, the greater the toxicity; however, some drugs can produce toxic reactions even when used in small doses.

Transient ischemic attack (TIA). A sudden, rapid onset of a focal neurologic deficit caused by a cerebrovascular disease. The deficit lasts less than 24 hours, reverting completely to normal.

Tremor. A rhythmic alternating movement.

Suggested References

Editors of Market House Books, Ltd. (1990). *The Bantam medical dictionary.* New York: Bantam Books.

Long, J. W.(1993). *The essential guide to prescription drugs.* New York: Harper Collins.

Meyer, M. E. (1993). *Coping with medications.* San Diego, CA: Singular Publishing Group.

APPENDIX

Abbreviations and Definition of Terms Associated with Medical Management

A, aa. of each

a.c. before meals

ad lib. as needed; as desired

ADD. average daily dose

ADR. adverse drug reaction

ADT. alternate day therapy

ALT hor. every other hour

aq. water

as.tol. as to

@B. at breakfast

@D. at lunch

@S. at supper

b.i.d. twice a day

b.i.n. twice nightly

cap. capsule

d. day

DNI. drug nutrient interaction

dr. dram

E.C. enteric coated

Elix. elixir

Fe. iron

g, gm. Gm. gram

HCL. hydrochloride

HCTZ. hydrochlorothiazide

h.s. at bedtime

I. iodine

IM. intramuscular

IV. intravenous

med. medication

mg. milligram

mm. millimeter

MOM. milk of magnesia

MVT. multivitamin tablet

N. nitrogen

NKA. no known allergies

NPO. nothing by mouth

NTG. nitroglycerine

o.d. every day

o.h. every hour

o.m. every morning

o.n. every night

os. mouth

OTC. over the counter

p.c. after meals

PCN penicillin

PO. by mouth

PRN. as needed; according to circumstances

q.d. daily

qh. hour

q.h.s. night at bedtime

q2h. every two hours

q.i.d. four times a day

q.o.d. every other day

qn. every night

qns. quantity not sufficient

qs. quantity sufficient

R$_x$. prescription

rept. let it be repeated

SE. side effect

SL. sublingual

s.o.s. if necessary

Speed. amphetamine

Sp gr. specific gravity

SQ. subcutaneous

SS. one-half

stat. immediately; first dose

Supp. suppository

Syr. syrup

tab. tablet

tmc. tincture

t.i.d. three times a day

t.i.n. three times a night

TPN. total parenteral nutrition

ung. ointment

ut dict. as directed

Vit. vitamin

xylo. xylocaine

ZOE. zinc oxide and eugenol

REFERENCES

Adler, L., Leong, S., & Delgado, R. (1987). Drug-induced stuttering treated with propranolol. *Journal of Clinical Psychopharmacology, 7*(2) 115–116.

Berry, W. R., Darley, F. L., Aronson, A. E., & Goldstein, N. P. (1974). Dysarthria in Wilson's disease. *Journal of Speech and Hearing Research, 17*(2) 169–183.

Brady, J. P., Burns, D., & Kuruvilla, K. (1978). The acute effect of haloperidol and apomorphine on the severity of stuttering. *Biological Psychiatry,* 13, 255-264.

Brady, J. P., Price, T .R., McAllister, T. W., & Dietrich, K. (1989). A trial of verapamil in the treatment of stuttering in adults. *Biological Psychiatry 25*(5) 630–633.

Brady, J. P. (1991). The pharmacology of stuttering: A critical review. *American Journal of Psychiatry 148*, 1309–1316.

Brumfitt, S. M., & Peake, M. D. (1988). A double-blind study of verapamil in the treatment of stuttering. *British Journal of Disorders of Communication, 23*, 35–40.

Burris, J. F., Riggs, M. C., & Brinkley, R. R. (1990). Betaxolol and stuttering. *Lancet 335*, 223.

Cocores, J. A., Dackis, C. A., Davies, R. K. & Gold, M. S . (1988). Propranolol and stuttering. *American Journal of Psychiatry. 143*(8), 1071–1072.

Costa, D. (1992). Antidepressants and the treatment of stuttering. *American Journal of Psychiatry, 149*(9), 1281.

Goldstein, D. M., & Goldberg, R. L. (1986). Monoamine oxidase inhibitor induced speech blockage. *Journal of Clinical Psychiatry 47*, 604.

Goldstein, J. A. Carbamazepine treatment for stuttering. (1987). *Journal of Clinical Psychiatry 48*(1), 39.

Harvey, J. E., Culatta, R., Halikas, J. A., Sorenson, J., Luxenberg, M., & Pearson, V. (1992). The effects of carbamazepine on stuttering. *Journal of Nervous and Mental Disease. 180*(7), 451–457.

Hays, P. (1987) Bethanecol chloride in treatment of stuttering. *Lancet 31*(1), 85270–85271.

Kampman, K., & Brady, J. P. (1993). Bethanecol in the treatment of stuttering. *Journal of Clinical Psychopharmacology, 13*(4), 284–285.

Kent, L. (1963). Use of tranquilizers in the treatment of stuttering: Reserpine, chlopromazine, meprobamate and atarax. *Journal of Speech and Hearing Disorders, 28,* 289–294.

Lozano, R. (1991). Comanagement of disordered speech motor control: The roles of the neurologist and the speech pathologist. In D. Vogel & M. P. Cannito, (Eds.), *Treating disordered speech motor control: For clinicians by clinicians* (Vol. 6, pp. 17–41). Austin, TX: Pro-Ed.

McLean, M. D. & McLean, A. (1985). Case report of stuttering acquired in association with phenytoin use for post-head-injury seizures. *Journal of Fluency Disorders, 10* (4) 241–255.

Murray, T. J. , Kelly, P., Campbell, L., & Stefanik, K. (1977). Haloperidol in the treatment of stuttering. *British Journal of Psychiatry 130,* 370–373.

Oberlander, E., Schneier, F., & Liebowitz, M. R. (1993).Treatment of stuttering with phenelzine. *American Journal of Psychiatry 150*(2) 355–356.

Posner, M. I., & Raichle, M. E. (1994). *Images of mind.* New York: Scientific American Library, HPHLP.

Prins, D., Mandelkorn, T., & Cerf, F. (1980). Principal and differential effects of haloperidol and placebo treatments upon speech disfluencies in stutterers. *Journal of Speech and Hearing Research 23*(3), 614–629.

Quinn, O., & Peachey, E. (1973). Haloperidol in the treatment of stutterers. *British Journal of Psychiatry, 130,* 379–433.

Restak, R. M. (1994). *Receptors.* New York: Bantam Books.

Rosenfield, D. B. (1988). Carbamazepine treatment for stuttering. *Journal of Clinical Psychiatry, 49*(1), 38.

Rosenfield, D. (1991). Pharmacologic approaches to speech motor disorders. In D. Vogel & M. P. Cannito, (Eds). *Treating disordered speech motor control: For clinicians by clinicians.* (Vol 6.) Austin, TX:Pro-Ed.

Styron, W. (1990). *Darkness visible: A memoir of madness.* New York: Random House.

Wells, O., & Malcolm, M. (1971). Controlled trial of treatment of 36 stutterers. *British Journal of Psychiatry, 119,* 603–604.

Zachariah, G. (1980). Verapamil in the management of stammering. *The Antiseptic 77,* 87–88.

INDEX